THE
CORE
CONNECTION

Go from Fat to Flat by Using Your Abs for a Total Body Workout

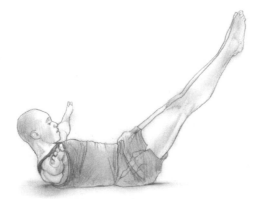

CHRIS ROBINSON

SIMON SPOTLIGHT ENTERTAINMENT
New York London Toronto Sydney

Note to Reader

This publication contains the opinions and ideas of its author. It is intended to provide helpful and informative material on the subjects addressed in the publication. It is sold with the understanding that the author and publisher are not engaged in rendering medical, health or any other kind of personal professional services in the book. The reader should consult his or her medical, health, or other competent professional before beginning an exercise program or adopting any of the suggestions in this book or drawing inferences from it.

The author and publisher specifically disclaim all responsibility for any liability, loss or risk, personal or otherwise, which is incurred as a consequence, directly or indirectly, of the use and application of any of the contents of this book.

S|S|E

Simon Spotlight Entertainment
A Division of Simon & Schuster, Inc.
1230 Avenue of the Americas
New York, NY 10020

First Simon Spotlight Entertainment hardcover edition January 2009

SIMON SPOTLIGHT ENTERTAINMENT and colophon
are trademarks of Simon & Schuster, Inc.

For information about special discounts for bulk purchases,
please contact Simon & Schuster Special Sales at 1-800-456-6798
or business@simonandschuster.com.

Designed by Jaime Putorti

Manufactured in the United States of America

10 9 8 7 6 5 4 3 2 1

Library of Congress Cataloging-in-Publication Data

ISBN-13: 978-1-4169-5084-4
ISBN-10:   1-4169-5084-2

CONTENTS

"I had a great body and didn't know it until I lost it. I don't know whose body this is; it's not mine. And I need to crawl out because it's just not working for me anymore.

—Christiane, 30

"I want to be here to see my daughters get married. If I don't start taking care of myself, I might not be around for that.

—Miguel, 33

"If I walk up two flights of stairs, I'm like, "Whoo! That was hard." It's just not convenient to live in a fat body.

—Angela, 30

"I'm a professional woman. I built a law practice from scratch. I handle myself pretty well, but I can't seem to get a handle on my weight. That I can manage my clients' problems but not my weight . . . that bothers me tremendously.

—Cindy, 44

"Sometimes in the morning, when I bend to tie my shoes, I can't breathe. I'm ready to change.

—Tim, 35

INTRODUCTION:
5 PEOPLE, 78 POUNDS, 6 WEEKS:
THE CORE CONNECTION DIFFERENCE

As a personal trainer, I help top athletes, celebrities, and executives get into the best shape of their lives. This book presents the same workout they use to achieve peak fitness. It also tells the story of five ordinary men and women who followed my program for six weeks—and achieved dramatic results.

I trained them myself, in San Diego, California—a challenging task, because of my weekly "commute." During the week I train in New York City, where most of my clients reside. On weekends I fly home to San Diego, one of the most beautiful cities in the world (and I've seen many when I travel with clients).

For six weeks, on most Thursday nights, I'd fly into San Diego, train the group Friday through Sunday, and then fly back to New York. While I was gone, they trained solo twice a week. These people had as much motivation and determination as any professional athlete or TV star I've trained, and in those 42 days, they changed their bodies and their lives. You'll meet them in the next chapter, but here's a mini-introduction.

Angela and Christiane. Best friends since grade school, these sharp, funny 30-year-olds still live across the street from each other. "We got fat together," Angela told me. "Now we want to get thin together."

Cindy and Tim. Overstressed, overweight, and overly fond of fast food, this couple wanted to get healthy for their boys. "We want to make a lifestyle change, not just diet and exercise for a few weeks and then go back to our old ways," Cindy said.

Miguel. My attorney and a good friend, Miguel is your typical hard-driving type: He works too much and moves too little. His body is the victim of his success, and he's ready to make time for exercise again.

These very different people shared a common goal: to take back their bodies. And they did. By our last class they'd lost a combined total of 78 pounds. Some had reached their goal weight; others were well on their way. All agreed they'd never experienced a more effective workout.

What makes my program different boils down to four words: *Train from your core.*

Work Beyond Your Abs

Let me guess: You hear the word "core" and picture washboard abs. You're partly right: The core includes the abdominal muscles. However, it also encompasses the 29 muscles in and around your trunk and pelvis, including those of the hips, buttocks, and lower back.

Or maybe you think core training involves hundreds of crunches or sit-ups. Nope. You can do crunches until you drop and still have a weak core.

Your core's main function isn't to look good in a bikini. It's to give your body strength, stability, and mobility. The core links your upper and lower body. When you bend to mop up a spill on your kitchen floor, or twist in your car seat to locate your seat belt, that movement originates in your core. A chain is as strong as its weakest link; your body is only as strong as its core.

A century ago, before cars and washing machines and supermarkets, folks got great core workouts: They farmed, chopped firewood, hung laundry on a line. Today most people begin their day in a car, spend most of it at a desk, and end it on a couch. Such sedentary behavior weakens core muscles. Your posture deteriorates; you slouch and slump. Your stomach bulges. Your lower back hurts. You're ripe for muscle injuries. The weaker your core, the less you move. The less you move, the more you weigh.

Athletes know the importance of core strength. Joseph H. Pilates, who almost a century ago created the brilliant training regimen that bears his name, knew it first. I was introduced to Pilates in 1999, and from my first lesson, I was blown away by its effectiveness. So blown away, in fact, that I became a certified Pilates instructor. From there I began to apply its principles to the workouts I created for my clients.

The Ultimate Total-Body Workout

My workout integrates the Pilates emphasis on core strength, muscle control, breathing, and correct posture into standard cardio and strength-training workouts. I also include basic Pilates matwork to help you find and feel your core muscles.

In my workout you don't just "do cardio" or "lift weights." You perform these workouts in a way that emphasizes alignment of the spine, muscle control, and—most important—contraction of the core muscles. You connect your core to every movement, hence the name of my program.

Core Connection offers two main benefits.

Dramatic increases in core strength and stability. These improvements benefit your posture, reduce back pain, reduce risk of muscle injuries, and enhance your ability to work out. They also enhance sports performance, whether you play tennis or golf, bowl or jog, ski or hike. A strong core improves your overall quality of life.

Increased calorie burn. When you activate your core muscles during cardio and strength training, you use more musculature. For example, when you perform a bicep curl, you don't simply work your bicep. You also work your buttocks, thighs, and abdominals. The more muscles you work, the more calories you burn. You build muscle faster. Body fat melts away. Your stomach flattens. Your lower body shrinks; your upper body gets lean and strong.

The Results Speak for Themselves

If five regular men and women can dramatically transform their bodies in six weeks, you can, too. After six weeks, if you have more weight to lose, simply keep going until you've reached your goal.

If you have 25 pounds or less to lose, six weeks should do it. For example, Tim had lost 15 pounds by Week 4. He did the group workouts *and* took challenging hikes with his sons. Midway through the program he also joined a baseball team. All this activity, combined with the diet, helped Tim's extra pounds melt away.

By the end of their six-week program, every group member pledged to continue the program. They'd learned that to reach and maintain a healthy weight, they'd have to work at it—every day. They'd already made the lifestyle changes required to get—and stay—fit and healthy.

"The program may be over, but Tim and I plan to continue on this path," Cindy said. "It would be hard not to. We feel so much better. We have more energy. In fact, we've planned another hike for this weekend, with our boys. We feel like we're setting a good example for them."

Train hard and commit to excellence, and you will change your body and perhaps your life. Yes, life does change when you get fit.

A few months back Angela e-mailed me. *Today Christiane and I hiked Cowles Mountain.* (By the way, Cowles Mountain is, at 1,592 feet, the highest point in San Diego.) *The last time I tried this, a few years ago, I got schooled by 85-year-olds and women carrying children. I couldn't make it all the way up. Today, I am proud to say, we made it to the top.*

I imagined Angela and Christiane struggling up that mountain, determined to take that peak. They deserve to feel proud. So does everyone else in the group. Their achievements are a direct result of their resolve. Each committed themselves to success and then did what it took to achieve it.

Make the same commitment. For the next six weeks, begin each day with that promise. Tell yourself, either silently or out loud: "Today I will do what it takes to get fit and healthy." Then *do what it takes.*

Your word is your bond to others, and to yourself. When you make a promise to a friend or family member, you keep it. Keep this promise to yourself. You'll be glad you did.

PART ONE

1
A GROUP INTRODUCTION

These days I train clients one on one. Only a few years ago, however, I taught 10 to 12 classes a week at two of the top health clubs in San Diego. I'd lead a Pilates or conditioning class in the morning and a kickboxing or functional training class later in the day. Some of my students were newbies; others had worked out for years.

I enjoyed teaching. I got fired up watching the newbies gain skill and confidence, or those who'd studied Pilates for years rededicate themselves to the craft every day. As I put together the group in this book, I found myself looking forward to rediscovering the camaraderie and energy that classes inspire.

Our first workout took place on a cool, breezy Saturday in January at Mission Bay Park in San Diego. I hadn't yet lined up a gym, so I told everyone to meet me at Tecolote Shores at this gorgeous state park. That's one of the benefits of my program—whether you use standard cardio and strength-training machines or portable equipment, like medicine balls and resistance tubing, you get an intense workout.

A few minutes before 11 A.M., Angela and Christiane pulled up, followed by Cindy and Tim, and Miguel. We stretched, took a brief warm-up jog, then got down to it. For the next 45 minutes, I coached them through a total-body workout that combined cardio, strength training, and the basic Pilates mat. None of them had exercised in years—or perhaps ever—but no one complained. No one left early. They were determined. I was impressed.

The first few weeks were tough on them—they were tired and sore. But as the weeks passed they grew leaner, stronger, and more confident. More than that, they became a unit. They groaned at me when I told them to hold a pose for 15 more seconds. They cheered each other on at every weigh-in. As I got to know them, they told me their weight, diet, and fitness stories. You're bound to find that at least one of them could tell yours.

Angela and Christiane

STARTING WEIGHT
Angela: 5'5", 162 pounds
Christiane: 5'8", 243 pounds

A petite brunette with doe eyes and gorgeous cheekbones, Angela is the friend of a friend of mine. She'd been heavy the last time we'd run into each other several months earlier, so she seemed like a perfect candidate for my group. I called, made my pitch, and asked if she wanted in.

"Definitely," she said. "Can I bring a friend?"

A few minutes before our first workout, Angela showed up with a tall, striking brunette—Christiane. "We've been best friends since second grade," said Angela, by way of introduction. "We grew up together."

"And got fat together," Christiane added. That's Christiane—she tells it like it is. Actually, they both do. Witty and outspoken, these two were definitely the comedians of the group.

As the weeks passed, I learned more about them. For example, both had athletic backgrounds. Now 30, Angela had played soccer and basketball and ran track in high school. "Lots of groups around here get together to play soccer or softball or other sports, but I'm too heavy to join them now—I'd kill myself," she said. "But I'd love to join one once I lose some weight." Christiane, also 30, began dancing at age six. "I still teach tap class, but I'm too heavy to perform now—I'd hurt myself."

In their midtwenties, they began to put on weight—together.

Angela's gain began with a breakup. "My boyfriend and I worked out five days a week and hiked and water-skied on the weekends," she said. "When we broke up, I went through a rebellious stage. I was like, I'm sick of working out." In six years she put on 60 pounds.

In college, Christiane taught 14 dance classes a week—modern, hip-hop, jazz—and performed most weekends. After graduation she slipped into a sedentary lifestyle and disastrous eating habits. "When I was little, my mom made me and my brother eat healthily," she recalled. "We couldn't have soda or sugary cereals or hamburgers and fries. But once I got a job and a car, it was fast food all the way." She tried crash diets a few times, but the 15 or 20 pounds she lost always returned.

Young and single, Angela and Christiane love to socialize, often meeting friends at a restaurant for dinner, then hitting a club. "All of our activities involve food or alcohol," Angela said. Now, "I'm learning that I don't have to drink or pig out to have fun."

While nervous about changing her behavior, Christiane did extremely well. Midway through the program she celebrated her thirty-first birthday. "No, I didn't have cake. I didn't even eat that much. We had this huge spread, and I had maybe two bites of something." (She drank alcohol, though, and paid for it the next morning. That's how you learn.)

Some of my clients remember the instant they vowed to get in shape for good. Angela and Christiane experienced more of a slow awakening.

"I felt a bit unhealthy," Angela said. "My cardiovascular health was not top notch. It got to the point where I wouldn't wear shoes with ankle straps. I was like, *Forget it. I do not want to be down there for 20 minutes buckling my shoes.*"

"I'd think, okay. Enough," Christiane said. "I'd think that every 10 pounds— *Wow, I gained another 10 pounds. This has got to stop.* Another 10—*Have to lose weight.* After a while I was like, *Eh, I'll worry about it next month.*"

Angela's goal weight was 135 pounds. Christiane didn't have a goal weight. "I'm not concerned with a number as much as how comfortable I am in my body," she said.

But Christiane did have a goal. "I want to dance and perform again. I miss it a lot," she said. "I have friends who perform. When I go to their shows, I think, *I wish that was me.* I hope that six weeks is long enough for me to change my lifestyle for good. Patience and I haven't ever been great friends, but it's time to get acquainted. I'm cautiously optimistic."

Miguel

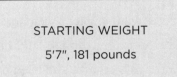

STARTING WEIGHT

5'7", 181 pounds

In 2006 I hired Miguel as my attorney, and we hit it off immediately. In 2006 I began to suggest—as casually as possible—that he might want to pay attention to his health. You know, lose a few pounds. Maybe check his cholesterol to see if his numbers were okay.

We were friends by then, and he knew I was right, so he took time out of one of his 12-hour workdays to get a checkup. A week later his doctor called, and Miguel gave me a full report. His total cholesterol was 270; his triglyceride levels, 420. The doctor wanted to write him a prescription for cholesterol-lowering medication. Miguel balked.

"I'm too young to take pills every day," he said. "I told him to give me a year—maybe I can get my numbers down with diet and exercise. What should I do?"

My advice was pretty basic. Walk or jog to raise his "good" HDL cholesterol and lower his "bad" LDL cholesterol. Swap his usual "breakfast"—a mug of coffee with powdered creamer and artificial sweetener—for a bowl of oatmeal. (Studies show that oatmeal helps lower cholesterol.)

"Great," Miguel said. Then, for the next year, he continued his unhealthy lifestyle. He ate salami-and-cheese heros at his desk, or took clients to his favorite Mexican restaurant for fat- and calorie-packed lunches. He did walk, though—from his car into his office.

I kept my mouth shut until I formed my group. Then, hoping I wouldn't offend my friend, I asked Miguel to join.

I shouldn't have worried. "I'm in," he said. "I've really let myself go. My pants don't fit. I have a belly. I'm only 33. I shouldn't look or feel like this."

In his youth, Miguel had been in prime shape. As a teenager in Mexico

City, he competed on a kickboxing team—he trained three or four hours a day—and earned his black belt at the age of 14.

At 19, he entered college, graduated, and then went on to law school, graduating in 2001. His martial-arts days were behind him, though, and he gained weight. Not a lot—maybe 12 or 15 pounds. Every so often he tried to lose weight and once dropped to 167 pounds on a crash diet of canned tuna. But he couldn't live on tuna alone—could anyone?—and the belly always returned.

After law school Miguel's life got even crazier. In 2006 he started his law practice. In 2005 he married Veronica and they started a family—Suzy was born in 2005 and Eliana in 2008. His pressure-cooker lifestyle didn't leave a lot of time to attend to his health.

Plus, he felt too guilty to spend a precious free hour working out. "My work demands long hours," he said. "I feel like if I go to the gym, I'm neglecting my family."

"Think of it another way," I said, explaining that taking time to work out didn't equal depriving his family of his attention. Rather, it ensured that he would remain with them, vital and healthy, for years to come.

Miguel agreed, but we knew he was in for a challenge: He'd have to make time to train with the group *and* exercise on his own twice a week, while making time for work and family. Hardest of all, he'd have to change his diet. "I love red wine, red meat, the Mexican food I grew up on," he said. "But I also love my family. I want to make this program the start of lifelong good habits."

Like me, Miguel's a straight talker, and he let me know, early on, that his goal wasn't to run marathons. "I don't watch sports. I don't do sports. I'd never ask a friend to go on a bike ride," he said. "I like to spend time with my daughters and go to the movies. My only goal is to live long enough to be a grandfather, and maybe a great-grandfather. If it takes me an hour a day to meet that goal, I'll give that hour."

That's good enough for me.

Cindy and Tim

STARTING WEIGHT
Cindy: 5'4", 200 pounds
Tim: 5'10", 235 pounds

Cindy, an attorney, had heard about my group from Miguel, her friend and colleague. Well-spoken, intelligent, and dynamic, she'd built her own law practice from scratch. Unfortunately, like many successful folks, she lived on a junk-food diet and sat at her desk for 10 to 12 hours a day. As a result of this unhealthy lifestyle, her weight was out of control.

Miguel gave Cindy my number and urged her to call me. During our talk, she asked if her husband Tim could join, too. I said sure.

"I guess I have no way out," she joked.

Of course, Cindy didn't want an excuse to continue her unhealthy lifestyle. In fact, as a parent, she could no longer justify it. Neither could Tim.

As a busy attorney, Cindy frequently worked late and rarely had time to cook. Neither did Tim, who was busy with the boys all day. As a result, their diet had degenerated into a steady stream of fast food and takeout. "I'll stop for Chinese on my way home, or we call for a pizza when I get there. Or we order from Applebee's or Outback and pick it up at the drive-through."

Cindy has struggled with her weight all her life and tried everything from prepackaged meal plans to medications to lose weight. Nothing had worked.

"Did you ever exercise?" I asked. She shook her head.

Tim's story was different. A former construction worker, Tim's intensely physical job had kept his weight under control. That changed several years ago when he quit his job to raise Timmy, four, and Charlie, now two. Tim often took the boys to a fast-food place for lunch. Although the boys weren't overweight, they were at serious risk.

"We've set a horrible example for our boys, and that has to change," Cindy said. "We had our kids late—I was 39 when Timmy was born—so every minute with them counts. The thought of us not being here for them because we chose to live an unhealthy life is unacceptable. We won't let that happen."

As the weeks passed, their dedication and effort continued to impress me. My workouts are simple, but they aren't easy, and both of them stepped up to the challenge.

When they first started the program, I was a little worried about them. Their fitness level was so far behind that I had to really modify the workouts and give them a lot of recovery time. Very quickly, though, they were able to keep up with the rest of the group. Cindy improved the most. The first day, she could barely perform some of the exercises. Now she can rise to the challenge. "This is the first program I can see myself sticking with for the rest of my life," she said. "I really enjoy it—and that's a lot coming from me because I hate to exercise. But I find your program so enjoyable."

Outside the group Cindy and Tim continued to challenge themselves. Their biggest challenge: preparing healthy meals at home. Bye-bye takeout and delivery, hello chicken, fresh vegetables, and brown rice.

"We cook together, or one of us bathes the kids while the other cooks," Cindy told me. "We've really pulled together to support each other. It's wonderful."

One Saturday morning, maybe two weeks into the program, Tim showed up for class, glowing. He told me that a few days before he'd taken a four-mile hike with his boys. It wasn't an easy hike, either—it was a switchback trail that goes up a mountain and up to a rock that overlooks the mountains of San Diego. "I haven't had a hike like that since my high school days, maybe 10 to 15 years ago. I am changing. I'm proud of Cindy, and Cindy is proud of me. But more important, we're proud of ourselves."

"Every morning Tim shows me his new muscles," Cindy said. "He is hilarious. Last night he made me work out even though it was an off day. We're loving this."

Now that you've met the group, let's get to work. In the next few chapters you'll learn all you need to know about the core principles of Pilates, the gear you'll need to start this program (hint: not much), and my nutritional guidelines.

" I'd heard about Pilates but didn't know much about it. I thought of it as an exercise for movie stars, not for people like me. But now that I'm actually doing it, I love it. I'd heard people who did Pilates say that there's nothing better for your body, and now I see why.

—*Cindy*

2
CORE PRINCIPLES

Pilates has its own language. Throughout this book, you'll hear certain words and phrases over and over again—"scoop," "Pilates stance," and "tuck chin to chest," for example. If you've tried Pilates in the past, you may know enough of the language to get by. If you're new to the Method, however, you may feel like a tourist in a foreign land.

This chapter is your phrase book. It illustrates and defines the most common Pilates concepts and expressions, which you'll need to follow the step-by-step exercises.

Joseph Pilates believed that his Method "develops the body uniformly, corrects wrong postures, restores physical vitality, invigorates the mind, and elevates the spirit." The six key principles, found throughout this chapter, are the foundation of the Pilates method. Try to integrate each of them into your workout. Don't limit their use to the matwork, however. You can use them in any exercise, and in everyday life.

The Scoop

To *scoop* is to draw the deepest layers of the abdominals—the transversus abdominis muscles—up and in. The purpose of scooping is to protect the spine. Scoop your abdominals, and you stabilize and align them. Let your abdominals hang out, and the spine has a lot of wiggle room, which can lead to back strain and injury.

Scooping is non-negotiable. If you don't have the scoop, your spine won't be in proper alignment, and you won't be able to perform the matwork safely and effectively. Nor will you engage your glutes.

The scoop isn't hard to learn: Whether standing, sitting, or lying

---

MAKING THE CONNECTION: LEARN ONE CONCEPT AT A TIME

When I teach Pilates, especially to a beginner, I choose one concept from this chapter and focus on it exclusively throughout our session. It's better to gain a solid understanding of one concept than a shaky idea of five or six.

I think this method is an easier way to grasp essential Pilates concepts, especially if you're new to Pilates, and I recommend you try it.

Before your workout, select one concept to focus on. It doesn't matter which—they're all important. If you want to zero in on the scoop, go ahead. If you'd rather focus on getting Pilates stance, that's great, too.

Once you've made your selection, focus on that concept, and that concept only, in each exercise. By the end of your session you'll have a better grasp of that concept in general as well as its role in each exercise.

The next time you do your matwork, choose another concept—maybe pressing your shoulders down and away from your ears, or chin to chest.

Work in this simple yet methodical way, and you're likely to progress quickly. After the first three weeks you'll have mastered the work's key components.

down, simply pull in your stomach until it takes on the concave shape of a bowl. The challenge is to maintain your scoop for the duration of an exercise, which can be tough even for me. Fortunately, the more you scoop, the faster you will develop core strength and stability. Follow my program faithfully, and before long you'll scoop without even thinking about it.

Pilates Stance

A key Pilates position, Pilates stance involves a slight outward rotation of the upper thighs, which helps stabilize the hips and pelvis and align the hips, knees, and ankles. Typically, however, Pilates stance is described in terms of the feet: heels together and toes apart, the feet assuming a slight V shape.

As your feet form the V, your powerhouse, or core, helps position them. Pilates stance originates from the powerhouse, and the V results from the powerhouse's activation of the inner thighs, the backs of the upper thighs (right below the glutes), and the glutes.

Whether you stand or lie on your mat, here's how to assume Pilates stance. First, bring your heels together and open your toes slightly, so that your feet form that V. Next, contract your glutes and squeeze the backs of your upper thighs together. You should feel the front of your thighs "wrapping" around to the backs of your upper thighs. Relax your feet and calves and scoop your stomach. Your thighs should be rotated slightly outward and your glutes contracted. Elongate your spine from your tailbone to the crown of your head, reach your crown and your spine up and away, and anchor your heels to the mat.

Pilates can transform your body, but it takes a focused mind to get results. Concentration is critical.

Concentration means focusing on the task at hand: your workout. Tune out all distractions: bills, what to make for dinner, or the argument you had with your child before school. Think of the shapes your body is making as you move and the sensations of your muscles as they stretch and work. Focus on contracting your glutes as you rotate your thighs into Pilates stance, pointing your toes, and elongating your fingers. When you can see your body moving correctly and feel your muscles do what you want them to do, you are in full concentration mode—and well on your way to a more toned physique.

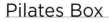

Pilates Box

Imagine a line drawing of a box on your torso. The first line runs vertically from your left shoulder to your left hip. The second runs vertically from your right shoulder to your right hip. The last two lines run horizontally from shoulder to shoulder, and from hip to hip.

That's the Pilates Box, which will help make sure that your shoulders and hips are aligned correctly. As you work, check your box often to make sure it's square. It shouldn't rotate to one side or get "squashed." If your box "collapses," you're twisting or leaning, which means you probably need to refocus and reposition yourself.

Chin to Chest

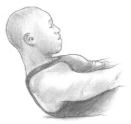

Proper alignment of the head and neck is important when you perform mat exercises that require you to lie flat while raising your head and extremities. Proper chin to chest positioning lets your abdominals do the work—which is what you want—rather than your neck, which will cause strain and discomfort.

When I ask that you "place chin to chest," raise your head above your breastbone and keep your eyes on your powerhouse, not on the ceiling. (Imagine holding a tennis ball under your chin against your chest.) Keep your shoulders back and away from your ears, too. If you're in the correct position, you should feel a stretch in the back of your neck, but no strain.

Don't bring your chin too far down on your chest or tilt your head back. This can strain your neck muscles and cause your abdominal muscles to bulge outward.

PILATES PRINCIPLE 2:
CENTER

Scoop. Draw your navel toward your spine. Suck in your stomach. No matter how you say it, in Pilates it is absolutely essential to work from your spine, abdominals, and glutes.

In Pilates, the energy for all movement begins in the powerhouse, or core, and flows outward to the extremities. You always work from your center, even if you're performing an exercise for your arms or legs. The strength in your core will "flow" to your extremities, giving them more power, range of motion, and control.

If you're just starting Pilates, patience is key. Practice and perfect the introductory matwork until you've developed the core strength required to tackle the intermediate mat. The difference you'll feel will be worth it.

PILATES PRINCIPLE 3: CONTROL

Concentration is about keeping your mind on your matwork, rather than on the events or worries of the day. Control is about actually using your mind to tell your body what to do. Think of your mind as your body's coach—encouraging it to lengthen here, contract there, reach toward the ceiling or the floor.

While control originates in the core, providing support for the spine, improving balance, and stabilizing the posture, it extends to the mind, creating discipline and focus. Your mind must control your body's every movement, especially at the beginning of each exercise, and as you move into the transitions. Performing the exercises with control also reduces the chances of injury.

PILATES PRINCIPLE 4: FLUIDITY

I wish you could see my Pilates teacher, Romana Kryzanowska, in action. You'd begin to appreciate the importance of fluidity—the graceful flow from one exercise to the next. Fluidity is the quality that makes Pilates so rewarding to perform and beautiful to watch.

Pilates exercises connect all parts of the body. When you perform them, you're not doing separate exercises, but one long, continuous activity, like a dance. It's Pilates' fluidity—its seamless flow, with no quick, jerky starts and stops—that challenges and tones your muscles and works your cardiorespiratory system.

That said, you will most likely not have this kind of flow your first time on the mat, or even your tenth. Don't fret. Just keep practicing, and you'll become in tune with the exercises. As you advance in your matwork, you'll achieve fluidity in your transitions, which are actually exercises in their own right. Once you can put the sequences together, you should be able to just flow right through. When you really know what you're doing, the introductory and beginner matwork should take eight to nine minutes; the intermediate mat, 18 to 20 minutes. Until then, work at your own pace, but give the work everything you've got.

Shoulders Down

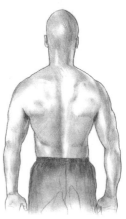

Many clients first come to me with their shoulders up around their ears. Some spent long hours hunched over their desks. Others habitually cradled a phone between their shoulder and ear. Still others acquired their crunched-up shoulders from poor workout habits, like lifting too-heavy weights. As a result, one of their shoulders was higher or lower than the other, which threw off their spine's alignment.

As you perform your matwork (and all the workouts in my program), use your latissimus dorsi muscles, or lats, to press your shoulders down and away from your ears. You'll protect your spine and reduce strain and discomfort to your neck. Proper shoulder alignment benefits you in your daily life, too. With your shoulders out of the way, your chest will have room to expand, allowing you to take fuller, deeper breaths.

PILATES PRINCIPLE 5: PRECISION

If control is the mind telling the body what to do, then precision is the body doing what the mind says. Precision is all about the appropriate placement of each body part, the alignment of each part to another, and the path of each motion.

But for your body to follow your mind's orders, you should already have a game plan. Only when your mind has retained the steps to each exercise, including transitions and breathing, can it tell your body how to move. Precision means remembering to reach your fingers away, to rotate your knee outward while also pointing your toes. Time, and paying attention to details, will bring precision to your routines. Eventually, this precision will become second nature.

Spine Position

In the lying-down position, the spine should be neither arched nor tucked. Arching puts a lot of pressure on the lower back and makes it difficult to activate the powerhouse. Tucking the back—flattening it so far into the mat that it lifts the hips off the floor—isn't desirable either, because it over-contracts the hip flexors.

Instead, press your tailbone into the mat while elongating your spine along the mat as much as you can. Then, focus on isolating your scoop without shifting your pelvis.

If your back's natural curves keep your lower back from touching the mat, press your tailbone into the mat, along with as much of your lower back as you comfortably can.

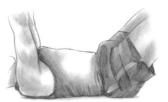

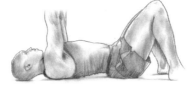

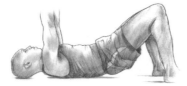

PILATES PRINCIPLE 6:
BREATH

In Pilates, as in all forms of physical activity, proper breathing helps the body exert itself and recover from that exertion. When you do Pilates (or any exercise), your muscles need more oxygenated blood to perform. So it's critical to breathe properly, taking full inhalations and exhalations and coordinating your breath with your movement.

Generally speaking, in Pilates, you inhale as you begin a movement and exhale as you execute it. As simple as this sounds, it can be challenging, even for me. When I perform a particularly strenuous movement, I really have to focus on staying relaxed and matching breath to movement.

As you become more familiar with the matwork, you will instinctively understand how to match breath to movement. But as the exercises get progressively more challenging, you may want to hold your breath. Don't let this happen. Pilates is about flow. As the movement should flow, so should your breathing.

"For the first two weeks, I did well. I made every workout, packed all my lunches and snacks. I was feeling good.

Then I got cranky. Not cranky like, "I want french fries." Cranky like a kid working up to a temper tantrum. It lasted maybe two days, but I got through it. I packed my workout clothes. Made my lunch and dinner. Found time during my workday to work out, shower, come back to work, and teach my tap class on Thursday night. It's a lot of effort, but it's totally worth it. I'm still here. I won't give up.

—Christiane

3
CORE PREPARATION

I start this chapter with Christiane's quote because it gets to the essence of what achieving peak fitness requires: pushing yourself.

I don't mean you need to do cardio until you're about to pass out, or lift weights that are clearly too heavy. To push yourself is to find out what you're made of, which requires both physical and mental stamina. One of the things I love most about sports is the exhilaration of reaching what you think is your limit—and exceeding it.

The first thing you can do to prepare for my program? Raise your expectations. Strive to make every workout better than the one before.

You may not always succeed, but that's not important. What's important is that you try. As you train, push harder. Find just a shred more to give.

Stay hungry. If you truly want to lose weight or get into the best shape of your life, you can. If you believe that success is within your grasp, and can hold onto that belief even when things get tough, you're halfway there.

As you begin to make that mental adjustment, let's discuss more practical matters, like the equipment you'll need to do my program at home and the principles I'd like you to keep in mind as you train. By the end of this chapter, you'll be ready to tackle the exercises in Part 2 and the workouts in Part 3. I'll be behind you every step of the way.

What You'll Need for Home Training

You may already have some of the equipment you'll need. But if you do need to buy it, you'll find everything at any Wal-Mart or Target, at minimal cost.

A cardio machine. You might already own a treadmill, elliptical trainer, stepper, or exercise bike. Cindy and Tim owned an elliptical, and they blew off the dust and used it for the first time in ages.

It doesn't matter which kind you have, as long as it's safe and in good repair. If you decide to purchase a cardio machine, you shouldn't have to spend more than a few hundred dollars. Treadmill, stationary bike, stepper . . . it doesn't matter. The best machine is the one you like the most (or dislike the least). If your budget is tight, you can always walk outside, or climb up and down a flight of stairs for the cardio portion of my workout. (If you opt to climb stairs, see page 241.)

Several sets of dumbbells. There are many choices—metal, chrome, coated with rubber. Any kind will do. I recommend that you buy three sets. If you're a woman, start with 5-pound, 8-pound, and 10-pound sets or 8-, 10-, and 12-pound sets. Lift them in the store to see which weights best match your current level of strength. If you're a guy, the in-store weight test is the best way to choose your weights.

If your budget allows, consider PowerBlocks. This adjustable dumbbell system is like several sets of dumbbells in one, which allows you to easily change the weight of the dumbbell by aligning a pin. (If you plan to train with a stronger partner—say, a husband or boyfriend—he can adjust for heavier weights.)

The SportBlock set (about $130) adjusts in 3-pound increments, from 3 to 24 pounds. You can purchase PowerBlocks at sporting-goods stores or online at www.powerblock.com.

An exercise mat. If you'll train on a carpeted surface, you don't need a mat. If not, a mat will give you a firm, comfortable surface on which to perform the Pilates matwork and some of the strength-training exercises. Make sure that the mat is long and wide enough to accommodate your entire body. You can also use a yoga mat or a large beach towel.

Resistance tubing/door attachment. Available in a variety of resistance levels (very light to heavy), resistance tubing allows you to perform a variety of strength-training exercises without dumbbells or machines. You'll use tubing for just one exercise, but you'll need two bands—one for now, and one to accommodate gains in strength.

The resistance (stretchiness) of the bands is coded by color. If you're a beginner, select the yellow tubing for now and graduate to green when you're ready. If you're at an intermediate level of fitness, opt for green and move up to red. Spend a few dollars more for the door attachment, too. It allows you to attach the tubing to any door for a safe, secure hold.

Workout clothing and footwear. Wear any clothing that allows you to observe the movements of your body as you train (especially important for the Pilates matwork). You don't need to run out and buy anything fancy—old tank tops and shorts are fine. Cross-trainers will give your feet the support they need during the cardio portion of your workout. If you plan to walk outdoors, it's a good idea to invest in good, supportive walking shoes, if you don't already own a pair.

Core Concepts to Train By

Don't "just do it"—do it right. True fitness isn't about how hard, how much, or how fast. It's about form. Whether you perform cardio, strength training, or Pilates, train consciously—don't drift away from the work. Check your form often, from the top of your head (frequently aimed toward the ceiling) to your toes (often placed in Pilates stance).

Concentrate on your core. Hold that scoop. Work from your abdominals, and work them deep. Scooping is absolutely crucial—it helps to stabilize and protect your spine, utilize your glutes for power, and keep your shoulders down. Focus on holding in your abdominals, and in time, the rest will fall into place.

Record your progress. Students take notes to help them perform better on tests. Athletes take notes, too, in the form of training logs. A training log is a chronicle of your progress, which you can use to set goals, assess strengths and weaknesses in your program, and sustain motivation. It's a record of where you've been, and a road map that will take you where you want to go.

You can use any log you like, or use the one I've provided on page 243. Photocopy a bunch, stick them in a binder, and fill one out during each training session. As you perform the workouts in Part 3, record the appropriate information: minutes of cardio completed, reps and sets of each strength-training exercise, and notes on the quality of your Pilates matwork. You'll be amazed at how quickly you improve.

MAKING THE CONNECTION: MINIMIZE MUSCLE SORENESS

For a week or so, everyone in the group let me know that their muscles felt a little stiff and sore. (I remember Tim asking, "Man, will we feel like this every day?") I told them what I'll tell you: This discomfort, called delayed onset muscle soreness, means you're getting stronger.

Basically, you're sore because you've challenged your muscles beyond their customary demands. The result: microscopic tears in muscle fibers, coupled with inflammation, which can make you wince when you walk down a flight of stairs or lift your arm to brush your hair. During the repair process, these tiny tears heal up, and the muscle gets stronger. Typically, the soreness is at its worst the first day or so following your first workout. "I was pretty sore the first week, but it was nice to know that I actually did still have muscles," said Angela.

If you experience mild soreness, hang in there. The discomfort typically fades in less than a week. Believe it or not, the best way to get rid of the soreness is to keep working out—but at a lower intensity level. Training circulates blood to the sore areas and carries the leftover waste products—a natural by-product of exercise—out of the muscles.

If you're in real pain, however, *do not work out*. Gentle massage helps, as does gentle stretching. If the pain lasts longer than about seven days or increases, however, call your doctor. You may have pulled or strained a muscle.

Your body needs water to perform virtually all of its functions, like digest food, eliminate waste and toxins, and carry nutrients to where they're needed. Water also helps build muscle and cushion and lubricate the joints, keeping the muscles elastic. It truly is the fluid of life.

That said, I know how hard it is to drink water throughout the day. Like you, I'm constantly on the run, and if I don't have a bottle of water in front of me, I tend to forget to drink it. But it doesn't take long for the body to become dehydrated. That's why it's important to drink enough water every day.

My personal goal is to drink up to two gallons of water a day, depending on my training schedule, but I don't expect you to. Drink as much water as you comfortably can—at least the recommended eight 8-ounce glasses a day. Sip a glass first thing in the morning to help cleanse the kidneys and detoxify your system. Don't try to chug down two or three glasses at a time, though. Your body can process only eight ounces every 30 minutes. More will wash right through you—and you'll be in the bathroom a lot.

Water hydrates your body and regulates its temperature during exercise, so sip throughout your workouts. How much depends on how much you sweat and how much water you lose. Since my workouts take less than an hour to complete, one 8-ounce bottle will typically be enough. But definitely drink more if you tend to perspire a lot, or train in warm weather.

Expect to get what you give. Though we live in a quick-fix, immediate-gratification world, anything worth having requires effort. In training, as in life, the more you give, the more you get back.

Think of each workout as a friendly competition against yourself, and strive to do better each season. Set realistic, achievable short- and long-term goals. Write them in your log. When you meet them, set new ones. Train consistently, and with determination, and you will develop a mental toughness that will push you to ever-higher levels of performance.

"It's been easier for Tim and me to change our diet than we thought—and we've made some pretty big changes.

We eat out less often, and when we do, we choose healthy alternatives: grilled rather than fried chicken, reduced-calorie entrées at chain restaurants like Applebee's. At home, we replaced white rice and white bread with brown rice and whole-grain bread. I used to bake cookies two or three times a week, plus cupcakes "for the kids" (or so I told myself). Now, I make sugar-free pudding or gelatin, and it's fine. The boys haven't missed their cookies and cupcakes—Tim and I ate most of them.

We also prepare dinner at home at least five times a week. That's a huge change—we used to order takeout almost every night. A few nights ago, I got home from work late. Tim had steaks with broccoli and brown rice waiting. Before, I would have stopped for Chinese or Mexican takeout on the way home. We also eat at the table with the boys instead of in front of the TV. We enjoy more family time and teach them manners at the same time.

We eat less, yet we're not hungry. We stop when we are full instead of until our plates are empty. We no longer plan our day around what to eat—I was surprised by how much we did that. Now, we eat to live, not live to eat. It's a cliché, but it's true.

—Cindy

4
CORE NUTRITION

I'm pretty basic when it comes to food and eating. I have no diet secrets to reveal. If there are foods that burn fat, I haven't heard of them. I don't categorize foods as good or bad. That said, you have choices, and some foods are better for a healthy, active body than others. If you want a quick fix, you've come to the wrong guy. If you want to lose weight and still eat food you enjoy, in satisfying portions, stick around. That I can do.

"I don't like the word 'dieting,'" Christiane told me at the beginning of the program. "That word makes me starvaceous."

I told her not to worry. I don't offer a "diet," just guidelines. If you follow them, and my fitness plan, I can virtually guarantee that those extra pounds will drop away.

Calories Count—
But You Don't Have to Count Them

No matter what diet you're on—low-fat, high-protein, vegetarian, the fad of the moment—calories matter. They always have, and they always will. I know that's not sexy, but it's true. Consume more calories than you burn, and you gain weight. Burn more calories than you consume, and you lose. That's it!

One client I'd worked with for years discovered this a few years ago. She was working out five days a week—taking my classes *and* running— and couldn't lose weight no matter what. She was even running marathons then, and those extra pounds were slowing her down.

One day, as she told me about her weight woes, she mentioned that she drank two glasses of red wine every night. That's easily 300 to 500 extra calories a day, depending on the size of the glass.

"Try cutting back to one glass, two or three times a week," I suggested. "See what happens."

Here's what happened: She lost 17 pounds in six weeks. Nothing else in her life changed—not the rest of her diet, not her activity levels.

If you need further proof that calories matter, look around. Despite the low-fat craze of the early 1990s and the more recent low-carb movement, a study conducted in 2006 by the federal Centers for Disease Control (CDC) found that 66 percent of Americans are overweight, up from 25 percent in the early 1970s. In the late 1970s, 15 percent of Americans were obese (30 percent above ideal body weight). Now, it's 32 percent.

We all know how this happened. You can't walk a block without passing a fast-food place, a coffeehouse, or a doughnut shop. Who even walks a block anymore? The root cause of the obesity epidemic: We consume too many calories.

In 1971, the average man consumed 2,450 calories, according to a 2004 study conducted by the CDC. In 2000, it was 2,618—an increase of 7 percent. Women's calorie intake rose from 1,542 to 1,877 calories in the same period, a 22 percent rise. (The current recommended intake for women is 1,600 calories a day.) For women, that extra 335 calories a day adds up to 122,275 calories per year—34 pounds' worth.

The CDC study also found that we consume most of those extra calories as refined carbohydrates—cheesy fries, sugar-laden lattes, chips, pasta, soda. Alarmed by the explosion of obesity, some cities, including New York City and San Francisco, require chain restaurants, such as Applebee's and Outback, to display calorie information on their menus or menu boards. Many restaurant chains nationwide already show calorie information to help customers think before they order a day's worth of calories at one meal.

So, yes, calories count. Still, and forever.

The Perfect Plate—Every Time

How many calories you need depends on your resting metabolism, which is influenced by your height, weight, age, and other factors. (To calculate your calorie needs, see page 45.) You don't need to do the math or log your daily calories unless you want to. Some of my clients do; they find that it keeps them honest.

But I do ask that you begin to eat *consciously*. To decide when and what to eat, instead of letting circumstances—a bad day, a late night, a lazy weekend—dictate your food choices. This mindfulness will reconnect you with the basics of healthy eating, which are all you need to lose weight.

For the next six weeks I ask that you take steps to raise your calorie consciousness. Monitor your portions. Scale back on high-fat foods as well as low-fat snacks or sweets, which tend to be high in calories. Limit or eliminate sugary soft drinks and fruit drinks; one University of North Carolina study found that Americans get an estimated *21 percent* of their daily calories from beverages. Since 1970, the number of calories adults get from drinks has doubled, and sodas, fruit drinks, alcohol, and other high-calorie beverages are fueling the obesity epidemic. Above all, pay attention to what you put in your mouth, and why.

Sure it's important to eat right. Because we're all so busy, though, it's equally critical that eating right be *easy*. So I came up with a simple way to create what I call the perfect plate—a meal that contains the right portions of the right foods. With the perfect-plate formula, you automatically build a healthy meal by choosing foods from six different segments. The result: a meal with nutritional balance, the appropriate amount of calories, and variety.

■ **Segment 1:** Lean protein, which includes fish, poultry, and lean cuts of red meat. Beans and soy foods are good sources of non-animal protein.

■ **Segment 2:** Eggs and dairy products, including egg substitutes and reduced-fat cottage and ricotta cheese, yogurt, and milk. (If you're a woman, this segment is particularly important, since you need calcium to build and maintain strong bones.)

■ **Segment 3:** Whole grains and whole-grain products that are gluten-free, which include the grains themselves and whole-grain breads, cereals, and pastas. I recommend that you consume only whole-grain products, with the exception of your once-a-week splurge.

■ **Segment 4:** Vegetables—you can't go wrong. I recommend that you limit starchy veggies such as corn, peas, and white potatoes. If you do eat them, stick to the correct portion sizes.

■ **Segment 5:** Fruits, which are rich in nutrients and fiber. There's no bad fruit, although I recommend that you eat sparingly of dried fruit, grapes, and pineapples, since they are especially high in natural sugars.

■ **Segment 6:** Healthy fats such as olive, canola, and safflower oils, fatty fish, such as salmon, tuna, and halibut, dark-green leafy vegetables, olives, and nuts and nut butters.

Generally speaking, combine one serving from Segment 1 *or* 2 (choose one) with one serving *each* from Segments 3–6, and you've got yourself a meal. Monitoring your portions is crucial, but don't worry about getting every Segment into every meal. The fat or fruit or grain you don't get in one meal, you can add to another.

One of my favorite meals is chicken or fish (Segment 1), brown rice (Segment 3), and grilled or roasted vegetables (Segment 4). As much as I travel, I've never had a problem ordering this meal, even if I had to ask the cook to prepare the meat or vegetables without butter, cheese, or creamy sauces.

What Fills My Perfect Plates

Some eating plans don't allow substitutions; the perfect plate formula encourages them. Each segment includes a wide variety of foods, so if you don't care for one or two, you're not bound to eat them because they're on your diet.

To inspire you to create your own perfect plates, I've listed five foods that fill my plate almost every day. You'll find them—and many more—in the Segment List on page 48.

Fish. I love salmon, and so do many people who don't care for fish in general. Salmon—any type of fish, actually—is low in calories and saturated fat and an excellent source of low-fat protein. Fatty fish like salmon, tuna, and halibut is rich in omega-3 fatty acids, which lower the buildup of fatty deposits in the blood, which can form clots that can contribute to heart disease.

Fish is no more difficult to prepare than meat or chicken. All I do is brush it with olive oil, throw it in a pan or baking dish, and cook it until it's cooked through and flaky. Some of my clients buy quick-frozen grilled fillets, which are as healthy and tasty as fresh-caught fish.

Chicken (white or dark meat). Many athletes and bodybuilders live on chicken breasts because they're high in protein and low in fat. Though the darker parts of the bird are higher in fat, I prefer them and eat them without guilt. One skinless chicken leg with a half cup of plain brown rice and a side of veggies is most definitely a perfect plate—a healthy, satisfying combination of protein, fat, and carbohydrate.

Brown rice. Only this grain's outer layer (hull) is removed during processing, which preserves its nutritional value. Brown rice is an outstanding source of complex carbohydrates, the body's preferred fuel, and is packed with vitamins, minerals, and phytonutrients (nutrients found in plants). I eat it almost every day and enjoy its sweet flavor.

Oats. Another staple of bodybuilders, this whole grain—loaded with vitamins, minerals, and health-enhancing phytonutrients—is as versatile as it is tasty. Plus, it's loaded with appetite-suppressing fiber, so a bowl in the morning staves off hunger for hours.

My clients get pretty creative with oatmeal. They stir in a tablespoon of low-fat fruit yogurt and a handful of berries, use oats to make pancakes or fresh muesli, a breakfast dish of Swiss-German origin. To make it, mix a half cup of rolled oats with a little grated apple, a tablespoon of seeds or chopped nuts, and a sprinkle of cinnamon.

Dark leafy greens. When you cut back on calories, it can be a challenge to get vital nutrients. Greens—spinach, kale, bok choy, Swiss chard, and collard and turnip greens—take up the slack. They're a good nondairy source of calcium. They're rich in vitamin A, in the form of the antioxidant beta-carotene, shown to help prevent age-related diseases like cancer. They're also a good source of the mineral magnesium (for bone and heart health) and the B vitamins folate and B_6 (also good for heart health). I sauté them in a drizzle of olive oil and add chopped garlic and cracked pepper.

Core Nutrition Guidelines

Using the perfect plate concept to build your meals primes you for success. The next step: Commit to these five simple guidelines for the next six weeks. They've worked for my clients; they'll work for you, too.

1. **Plan tomorrow's menu today.** You know what's on your plate tomorrow, schedule-wise. Use that information to plan what's on your plate, literally. Each day for the next six weeks, take five minutes to jot down tomorrow's menu. Some of my clients use a small notebook kept just for that purpose.

Some questions to think about: Do you have time for a sit-down breakfast, or does a grab-and-go meal better suit your schedule? If you bring lunch, what will you pack, and do you have it in the house? If you have a business lunch, do you know where you'll eat and what healthy menu items are available? Will you cook dinner, or order out? If you cook, will you eat what your family eats, or make your own meal? If you order out, what healthy choices will you make? If you ask these questions today, you're sure to succeed tomorrow.

2. Eat breakfast every day. Breaking your night's fast revs your metabolism and helps prevent the night munchies that can wreck your diet. In a study conducted by the National Weight Control Registry, a database of nearly 3,000 people who have kept off 30 or more pounds for at least a year, 78 percent of those surveyed said they ate breakfast daily.

Before Miguel started the program, his "breakfast" was a mug of coffee with nondairy creamer and artificial sweetener. "Now," he said, "I have a bowl of oatmeal with a teaspoon of honey—I don't use artificial sweeteners—and green tea. I also drink a lot of water. That holds me until lunch."

Oatmeal is a filling, tasty start to the morning. You might also opt for a tablespoon of natural peanut butter on a piece of whole-wheat toast, or a smoothie with low-fat yogurt, fresh berries, and skim milk. Keep a box of whole-grain cereal and a quart of skim milk in the office refrigerator and eat at your desk.

3. Practice portion control. It's virtually impossible *not* to lose weight when you eat healthy and your portions are spot-on. If you've never measured your food before, break out the measuring cups and spoons and invest in a food scale. Using them isn't as time-consuming as you'd think, and you'll be surprised—at times, shocked—to learn how much cereal, or peanut butter, or beef, you used to consume. After a few weeks you can start to eyeball your portions. The guide on pages 45–46 can help.

4. **Eat small, but often.** If you eat three square meals a day, break them into four to six smaller meals of 200 to 300 calories each, depending on your calorie needs. Research suggests that older women burn fat from large meals less effectively than younger women, but both burn fat from small meals equally well. So eating smaller amounts more frequently may make it easier to control your weight, especially if you're over 40. For 20 tasty mini-meals, see pages 57–59.

5. **Upgrade your carbs.** You already know that bagels, pasta, and other foods made with white flour or sugar tend to pack weight on. Enjoy them during your once-a-week splurge, which I'll discuss in a minute. The rest of the time stick to correct portions of healthy complex carbohydrates—whole-grain breads, cereals, and pastas, oatmeal (whole oats, not the instant varieties), brown rice, and sweet potatoes (one small one or half a large one).

6. **Be honest with yourself.** These days there's so much nutrition information out there that it's hard not to know when you make less-than-healthy food choices. My older brother, Marc, is a perfect example. I love him, but his eating habits drive me nuts. He thinks fruit punch is healthy because it has 10 percent fruit juice in it. He buys the type of sugary corn-pop-type cereal kids eat. Once, when he was out of town, I house-sat for him and raided his refrigerator. I didn't throw out his food—I just put my healthy choices next to his stuff. When he came back, there was fresh-squeezed orange juice next to his fruit punch, wheat bread by his white bread, sliced deli turkey next to his bologna.

He appreciated my gesture and even ate the healthy items I bought.

But my refrigerator makeover didn't stick. Recently I went home to see my dad in Houston and then went to Marc's house. What was in his refrigerator? Fruit punch, white bread, and bologna.

My point is, he knows which foods are healthy and which aren't, and so do you.

Splurge Once a Week

Sticking to my program requires discipline. But from time to time we all need to eat what our hearts desire rather than what our bodies require. That's why I want you to splurge once a week.

This built-in cheat actually helps you stay on track. It's easier to stay strong and eat healthfully when you know that on Wednesday, or Saturday, you get to eat something you truly love. Deprivation leads to cheating and binges. Planned indulgence fosters balance.

So that you continue to meet your goals, however, let's define "splurge": 400 calories over your normal allotment. My clients usually plan their cheats for the weekend—a Saturday-night dinner, say, or a Sunday brunch. Spend those extra calories on whatever you wish, such as a scoop of ice cream after dinner, a fast-food burger for lunch. Just choose your splurge carefully. Don't blow it on something you don't truly love.

Make sure you consume only 400 calories' worth, too. Measure out the two cups of cheese puffs and put them in a bowl. Take five chocolate-chip cookies out of the bag, then put the bag away. (Better yet, buy a single-serving size.) If you're dining out, ask for half the appetizer or entrée to be boxed in the kitchen. My clients and I do that all the time, and I find it's typically no big deal.

Good food is one of life's pleasures. When you have that pizza or hot-fudge sundae once a week, it will taste that much sweeter, because you will truly appreciate it.

Troubleshoot to Stay on Track

Office birthday parties. Dining out. Vacations. The holidays. The world around you, your very life, conspires to derail your diet at every turn.

That doesn't mean you have to be derailed. Sure, you'll falter sometimes. You're human! But if you make healthy choices most of the time, you'll come out ahead. Use this situation-by-situation troubleshooting guide to avoid the most common danger zones.

DINING OUT

■ Fill up on a clear, broth-based soup or a salad before your meal. Ask for the dressing on the side. Dip your fork into the dressing first, then spear the lettuce and veggies.

■ Most restaurants accommodate health-conscious customers. Politely request a side salad instead of fries, or an omelet made with egg whites.

■ Split an entrée with your dinner partner and order a salad and extra vegetables.

■ Ask the waiter to take the bread basket away, or place it on the other side of the table.

Weekends

■ Make it a point to eat a healthy breakfast—a veggie-stuffed egg-white omelet with whole-grain toast, or a fresh fruit salad or smoothie. You have more time to cook a healthy morning meal, and you'll probably eat less the whole day.

■ Don't go hungry to "save calories" for a big dinner out. Follow the dining-out tips on page 41.

■ Cut back on your alcohol intake—one glass of wine with dinner or two light beers at a party. The more you drink, the less likely you are to stick to your diet.

Office birthday parties

■ Sing "Happy Birthday," then slip back to your office before the first slice of cake is cut.

■ Offer to cut the cake, or pass it out. No one will notice you're not having a slice.

■ Have a *small* slice of cake if it's truly spectacular. Then scale back on lunch or dinner, or perform an extra 20 minutes of cardio.

The holidays

■ Eat before you attend a holiday party. You'll be less likely to fill up on high-calorie Christmas cookies and appetizers.

■ If you're invited to a dinner party, skip the cocktail hour and arrive at mealtime.

■ Don't skip a meal before a big holiday blowout. You risk gorging on sweets and other high-calorie fare.

■ Limit or avoid alcohol, which lowers your inhibitions about sticking to your diet.

■ If you're cooking a holiday meal, streamline it. Serve raw veggies with dip for an appetizer, a low-fat main course with one or two vegetables, and a fruit salad for dessert.

Vacations

■ Work physical activity into your leisure time. Pack your running shoes so you can jog along the boardwalk, or book a hotel with a gym.

■ If your hotel room has a minibar stocked with chocolate and chips, refuse the key.

■ Limit your alcohol intake. Have one piña colada or strawberry daiquiri poolside, then switch to water or club soda. Better yet, skip alcoholic beverages entirely.

■ If you're going to indulge, do it somewhat healthfully. Splurge on lobster tail—with lemon, no butter—or a jumbo shrimp cocktail.

OVERVIEW: CORE NUTRITION

• Design your meals with the segments on pages 48–55. In general, to make a meal, combine 1 serving from Segment 1 *or* 2 (choose one) with 1 serving *each* from Segments 3–6.

• Track portions and servings. Use measuring cups and a diet scale at first, then graduate to eyeballing portion sizes. If you tend to eat when you're bored or stressed, or if you nibble as you cook, consider keeping a food log.

• Read labels to determine the number of calories in a serving. You'll be less likely to consume more than a serving of foods you'll regret eating later.

• Eat every three to four hours, for a total of four to six 200- to 300-calorie meals a day. At the minimum, eat breakfast, lunch, a midafternoon snack, and dinner. If you eat breakfast very early, have a snack before lunch. Have a post-dinner snack if you need one.

• Plan your meals a day in advance, and never skip a meal.

• Consume several servings of calcium-rich foods a day. These include low-fat or nonfat dairy products or leafy greens.

• Drink eight glasses of water a day to flush away toxins and discourage water retention.

• "Cheat" once a week with ice cream, pizza, chips . . . whatever. Indulge up to 400 calories over your usual allotment.

How Many Calories Do You Need?

I dread when people ask me this question, because they usually are dissatisfied with my answer. And my answer is: It depends. How old are you? How active are you? How much of your body is muscle as opposed to fat? There are so many variables.

I think most people know when they consume too many calories, and I see no reason to burden you with complicated formulas that are never exact. Eat just when you're hungry, and stop when you're full (as opposed to stuffed). However, when people insist on a number, I give them this formula that gives a rough estimate of how many calories you need daily to maintain your *current* weight:

Multiply your current weight in pounds by:

- 11 if you get little or no exercise

- 13 if you get 30 minutes of exercise four or more days a week

- 15 if you get 60 minutes of exercise five or more days a week

For example, if you currently weigh 170 pounds and you don't exercise, multiply 170 x 11, which equals 1,870 calories. This is the number of calories you would need to consume to *maintain* your current weight.

Of course, you may want to reduce your weight. To lose a pound a week, subtract 500 calories from your current daily calorie requirements (1 pound = 3,500 calories). As you lose weight, you'll need to further reduce your daily calories to maintain weight loss.

Go On Portion Control

Fast-food places push value menus. Restaurants serve meals on plates as big as hubcaps. No wonder most people have lost sight of what an actual serving looks like. This guide can help.

FRUITS AND VEGETABLES	**ONE SERVING LOOKS LIKE . . .**
1 cup salad greens	a baseball
1 medium fruit	a baseball
1 baked potato	a computer mouse

GRAIN PRODUCTS	**ONE SERVING LOOKS LIKE . . .**
1 cup cereal flakes	your closed fist
1 bagel	a hockey puck (yes, that small)
$\frac{1}{2}$ cup rice, pasta, potato	the amount that would fit in an ice-cream scoop

DAIRY	**ONE SERVING LOOKS LIKE . . .**
1 $\frac{1}{2}$ oz cheese	4 stacked dice
$\frac{1}{2}$ cup ice cream	half a baseball
1 cup milk, yogurt	your closed fist

PROTEINS	**ONE SERVING LOOKS LIKE . . .**
3 oz meat, fish, poultry	a deck of cards
3 oz fish (grilled, baked)	your checkbook
2 T peanut butter	a Ping-Pong ball

FATS	**ONE SERVING LOOKS LIKE . . .**
1 t oil	your thumb tip

Lots of people eat to soothe boredom, loneliness, or stress. But the bottom line is, the only real reason to eat should be to satisfy physical hunger. Food is fuel for the body—no more, no less. If your emotions drive your food intake, you must confront those emotions. You must feel them, analyze them, and then decide whether they are a valid reason to eat.

Christiane identifies herself as an emotional eater. Once she began to analyze how she felt before she ate, rather than after, she made smarter choices.

"I think my weight was the effect of my depression, not the cause," she said. "What this boils down to is, I didn't get depressed because I was overweight. I was overweight because I was depressed.

"I also think I was eating for the lethargy you feel after you eat a huge meal. When you're stuffed and sleepy, you lose focus on the very things that drove you to eat in the first place."

"Eating to fuel your body is a completely different mindset," said Christiane. She is learning to separate the process of eating from the emotions it stirs up. "Now, when I want a cookie, I try to figure out why," she said. "I'm feeling something—bored, stressed, overtired, angry, worried. So far, what works for me is to eat with my head, not my heart."

Thinking before she eats isn't second nature for Christiane. It takes as much discipline as remembering to engage her core during her workout. But she's getting there.

So can you. If you can see food for what it is—energy for the body rather than sustenance for the soul—then you can break its hold over your life. You might find it helpful to keep a food journal. Nothing too complicated—just jot down how you feel every time you eat. You'll learn to identify when you're eating to feed your heart rather than your body.

Perfect Plate Menu Planning Segments*

Segment 1: Lean Protein

Women: 5 1-oz Segments a day

Men: 6 1-oz Segments a day

FISH

All finfish, including:

- Catfish

- Flounder

- Haddock

- Salmon

- Sea bass

- Swordfish

- Trout

- Tuna

---

*A Note on Calorie Needs

Everyone's calorie needs are different. You may need to alter your segments, based on your age, sex, and physical activity level. Based on federal guidelines, women should consume 1,600–2,400 calories per day; men, 2,000–2,800 calories per day. The older and less active you are, the fewer calories you need. To calculate your personal calorie needs, log onto www.healthfinder.gov/docs/doc08652.htm.

All shellfish, including:

- Clams

- Crab

- Lobster

- Mussels

- Oysters

- Scallops

- Squid (calamari)

- Shrimp

Canned fish, including:

- Anchovies

- Tuna

- Sardines

POULTRY

- Chicken or turkey, white or dark meat, skin and all visible fat removed

- Lean ground chicken or turkey

MEAT

■ Lean cuts of beef, ham, lamb, pork, veal

■ Game (such as rabbit or venison)

■ Lean ground meats such as beef, pork, and lamb

■ Deli meat, lean cuts (turkey, ham, chicken, roast beef—no bologna or liverwurst)

BEANS AND LEGUMES ($\frac{1}{4}$ CUP SERVING = 1 SEGMENT)

■ Black beans

■ Chickpeas

■ Kidney beans

■ Lentils

■ Navy beans

■ Pinto beans

■ Soy foods

■ Soy burger or hot dog, 1

■ Soy cheese, 2 oz

■ Soy milk, 8 oz

■ Soy nuts ($\frac{1}{4}$ cup serving = 1 Segment)

■ Tofu or tempeh

Segment 2: Eggs and Dairy

Women: 3 Segments a day

Men: 3 Segments a day

1 Segment equals:

- Whole egg, 1 (maximum of 2 whole eggs per day)

- Egg whites, 3–4 per serving

- Egg substitutes, $\frac{1}{3}$–$\frac{1}{2}$ cup per serving

- Reduced-fat yogurt, 1 cup

- Reduced-fat cottage cheese, 1 cup

- Reduced-fat milk (skim or 1 percent), 1 cup

- Cheese, light or nonfat, 2 oz

- Fat-free ricotta, $\frac{1}{3}$ cup

Segment 3: Gluten-Free Whole Grains*

Women: 4 1-oz Segments a day

Men: 6 1-oz Segments a day

1 Segment equals:

- Barley, $\frac{1}{2}$ cup cooked

- Brown rice, $\frac{1}{2}$ cup cooked

- Oatmeal, $\frac{1}{2}$ cup cooked

---

*Natural-foods stores carry less common but very tasty whole grains—such as buckwheat, millet, quinoa, and rye, as well as raw oats—and also breads and wraps made from them.

■ Whole-grain pasta, $\frac{1}{2}$ cup cooked

■ Whole-wheat bread, 1 slice

■ Whole-grain ready-to-eat cereal, 1 cup

■ Whole-grain cooked cereal, $\frac{1}{2}$ cup

■ Whole-wheat pita or wrap, $\frac{1}{2}$ wrap

Segment 4: Vegetables

3 Segments a day (women)

4 Segments a day (men)

1 Segment equals 1 cup raw or cooked vegetables and 2 cups of raw leafy greens

■ Artichoke (1)

■ Asparagus

■ Avocado ($\frac{1}{4}$)

■ Beets

■ Bell peppers

■ Broccoli

■ Brussels sprouts

■ Cabbage

■ Carrots

■ Cauliflower

- Celery

- Cucumbers

- Eggplant

- Green beans

- Leafy greens: collard greens, kale, mustard greens, romaine lettuce, spinach, Swiss chard, turnip greens

- Mushrooms, any variety

- Onions

- Potatoes

- Squash, any variety

- Sweet potatoes or yams

- Tomatoes

Segment 5: Fruits

1.5 Segments a day (women)

2 Segments a day (men)

1 Segment equals:

- Apple, banana, pear: 1 small or medium, $\frac{1}{2}$ large

- Berries (strawberries, blueberries, raspberries, etc.): 1 cup whole, $\frac{1}{2}$ cup sliced

- Citrus fruits (orange, grapefruit): 1 whole orange, $\frac{1}{2}$ grapefruit

- Grapes: $\frac{1}{2}$ cup (about 15 grapes)

- Kiwifruit: 1 medium

- Melon (cantaloupe, honeydew, watermelon): 1 cup chunks

- Papaya: $\frac{1}{2}$ cup, cubed

- Plums: 1 medium

Segment 6: Healthy Fats

3 Segments a day (women)

4 Segments a day (men)

- Avocado: $\frac{1}{4}$ fruit

NUTS & SEEDS

1 Segment equals:

- Almonds: 12

- Cashew nuts: $\frac{1}{2}$ oz

- Pistachio nuts: 24

- Peanuts: $\frac{1}{2}$ oz

- Pumpkin seeds: $\frac{1}{2}$ oz, hulled

- Sunflower seeds: $\frac{1}{2}$ oz, hulled

- Walnut halves: 7

- Nut butters: 1 tablespoon

OILS

1 Segment equals 1 teaspoon

- ■ Olive oil

- ■ Canola oil

- ■ Safflower oil

Four weeks into the program, Angela broke her diet. Accompanied by Christiane, who'd witnessed it, she told me about it the next day. "I feel like I have to confess," she said.

I asked if it was a slip-up or a full-blown binge.

"Well, if a binge means going to a restaurant opening where the food is free, and eating chocolate cake, carrot cake, and cheese-cake—"

"And appetizers—" added Christiane.

"Then, yes, I binged," Angela said.

"*Ange*," I said, and shook my head.

"I've been so good," Angela groaned. "It was just one night."

Then she told me what happened. A friend of Christiane's had opened a new restaurant and invited the girls. "I was like an addict," Angela admitted.

"She went psycho over the food," Christiane added.

"At that point I had not eaten salt, sugar, oil, butter, nothing," said Angela. "I was reeling. I actually stole someone's chocolate cake."

Apparently, Angela had ordered a slice, but the restaurant had run out by then. One of them spied a whole cake at a table across the restaurant. The girls knew the people at the table.

"So Christiane said, 'Go over. Ask if you can have a bite,'" Angela said. "I was like, 'That's crazy.' She said, 'Just do it.' I said, 'Okay.' So I walked across the restaurant with my fork, went up to their table, and said, 'So, I noticed you guys got the chocolate cake. Do you mind if I have a bite?'"

Her friends told her to take the whole cake; they were stuffed. So Angela carried it back to her table.

Thankfully, Angela didn't do as much damage as she could have. "I took maybe five bites," she said. "Also, I had a few bites of carrot cake and one bite of cheesecake."

I asked her how she felt. "Hungover," she replied. "I woke up with a headache, and I was nauseous."

But here's the good news: Angela did exactly what you're supposed to do after a binge. First, she showed up for her workout. Second, she returned to her diet. Even though she'd slipped up, Angela was right back on track—and that's what counts.

Like Angela, you might hit a few snags while on the program. If you mess up, don't deny that it happened. Figure out *what* happened. Determine the chain of events and emotions that led to your slip-up. Write it all down: what you ate, how you felt before and afterward. Go right back to your normal eating plan, too. Don't skip breakfast or starve yourself—your physical hunger will trigger another binge.

After you've analyzed the situation and figured out what happened, let it go. It's in the past. Guilt won't get you anywhere. Learn from it and move on.

20 Tasty Mini-Meals

Many of my clients eat five or six 250- to 300-calorie mini-meals every two or three hours, including before or after a workout. By eating every several hours, their blood sugar stays steady and they never feel hungry. Women over 40 add that mini-meals seem to control bloating and weight gain.

I favor grazing, as long as you keep your mini-meals truly mini. If they start to inch toward maxi, you may eat more calories than you need and actually gain weight.

I asked my clients who favor grazing throughout the day for a few of their favorite mini-meals. Try one, try them all.

Sweet minis

■ Top a whole-grain frozen waffle with 1 tablespoon natural peanut butter and 1 medium sliced banana.

■ Mix ½ cup cottage cheese with ¼ cup whole-grain cereal; top with ¼ cup fresh berries.

■ Stir 1 small handful sliced natural almonds into 1 cup low-fat fruit yogurt.

■ Peel a medium banana, then split it lengthwise. Spread with 1 tablespoon natural peanut butter and drizzle with 1 tablespoon chocolate syrup.

■ Spread 1 slice whole-grain bread with 1 tablespoon natural almond butter and 1 teaspoon honey or sugar-free jam.

■ Spoon a dollop of low-fat fruit yogurt on ½ cup fruit salad; top with 1 tablespoon chopped walnuts.

Savory minis

■ Sauté 2 egg whites in a nonstick pan, top with $\frac{1}{2}$ ounce reduced-fat cheese, and wrap in a small whole-wheat tortilla.

■ Stuff half a whole-wheat pita with 3 ounces smoked turkey breast and a few leaves of lettuce or spinach. Drizzle with olive oil and vinegar.

■ Top 1 cup mixed greens with 3 ounces grilled chicken; drizzle with 1 tablespoon nonfat dressing, and wrap in a whole-wheat tortilla.

■ Top a whole-grain English muffin with $\frac{1}{4}$ cup pasta sauce and 1 ounce part-skim shredded mozzarella. Pop it under the broiler until the cheese melts.

■ Combine $\frac{2}{3}$ cup cooked brown rice with $\frac{1}{2}$ cup canned black beans and 1 tablespoon lime juice; top with $\frac{1}{4}$ cup low-fat cheddar. Microwave for 1 minute on medium.

■ Mix 2 ounces canned tuna (packed in water; drained) with 2 tablespoons fresh, mashed avocado. Scoop onto 10 bagel chips.

■ Microwave a medium potato for 10 minutes on medium setting. Slice open lengthwise and top with 2 tablespoons salsa and $\frac{1}{4}$ cup shredded reduced fat cheese.

■ Spread 2 tablespoons fat-free black bean dip, $\frac{1}{4}$ cup shredded reduced-fat cheese, and 2 tablespoons salsa on a whole-wheat tortilla. Bake for 10 minutes in a 400-degree oven. Add $\frac{1}{4}$ cup shredded romaine. Roll up and enjoy with extra salsa on the side.

■ Microwave a whole-wheat pita for 1 minute on medium. Cut into triangles and spread with 2 tablespoons store-bought hummus.

■ Spread $\frac{1}{2}$ small whole-wheat pita with mustard; top with 2 thin slices of deli-sliced turkey breast, cucumber, and sliced tomato.

■ Top $\frac{1}{2}$ whole-wheat English muffin with 1 ounce reduced-fat mozzarella, green bell pepper, and tomato slices.

■ Top 1 slice whole-wheat toast with 1 scrambled egg and 1 slice turkey bacon.

■ Layer 2 slices deli-sliced chicken breast or ham, tomato slices, and lettuce on a whole-wheat tortilla. Top with a thin slice of avocado and 1 tablespoon salsa.

PART TWO

"My wife used to do Pilates, so I always thought of it as a women's thing. But when we started to train with Chris, I saw that Pilates is for everyone—old, young, women, men. I also saw how practical it is. You can do it at home, and all you need is a towel to lie on. The movements feel so relaxed, but at the same time, you can feel your muscles working really hard.

I'm not a coordinated guy, but I don't have to be—I still get a great workout. All I have to do is focus on using my core. This workout is so quick and simple, but at the end I feel great.

—*Miguel*

5
MATWORK

If you're trying Pilates for the first time, you're probably wondering what to expect—I know I did. Before you get started, let me walk you through the elements that make up the exercises in this section.

Illustrated, step-by-step instructions guide you through each exercise. Before you try an exercise, study each illustration carefully, and pay special attention to the positions of the spine, neck, and shoulders.

Transitions—positions that end one exercise and take you into the next—are as important as the exercises themselves. They're in boldface italics at the end of each exercise's final step.

Modifications adjust an exercise to make it more or less challenging; these are helpful if you have a physical limitation (such as a back, shoulder, or knee injury) or need to build your strength, endurance, or flexibility. You'll find the modifications, if any, after the step-by-step instructions.

Bulleted cues to the essential Pilates principles (concentration, control, center, fluidity, precision, breath) help you incorporate these ideals into each exercise.

Check your form illustrations help you correct errors most beginners make. Since I can't be there to move your knee or shoulders into the correct position, these illustrated "don't"s do the coaching for me.

Step-by-step illustrations in miniature help you understand the progression of the exercise at a glance so you don't get lost. Refer to them as you progress through your workout.

Tips for Success

To get the most out of your Pilates workout, you must use your mind to control your muscles and really study your body as it moves. Especially during your first few sessions, work at the speed at which you can control your movements. If you think you're moving *too* slowly, don't worry. You can't pay too much attention to form and technique.

Though you may feel awkward, your body is undergoing a transformation. After the first week, expect to stand taller and feel stronger, more flexible, and more energized.

Follow these tips, too. They'll make your Pilates practice productive and enjoyable.

■ Wear clothing that is comfortable, but not overly roomy. Baggy sweats or T-shirts are fine for jogging, but they hide your body, and with Pilates you need to be able to study yourself as you work.

■ Work in bare feet or treaded socks, so you can flex your feet freely.

■ To protect your spine, work on a mat, carpet, or blanket. In a pinch, several large towels will do.

■ If an exercise causes you discomfort or pain, stop. Pilates is about listening to your body. *Never* try to "work through the pain."

■ Take as long as you need to master the Introductory and Beginner matwork. Move on to the Intermediate matwork only when you can perform the Beginner matwork—including the transitions—smoothly and with correct form.

INTRODUCTORY MAT

THE HUNDRED

Stimulates circulation • enhances breathing

REPETITIONS
50–100 arm pumps (5–10 full breath cycles)

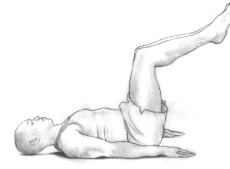

STARTING POSITION

Lie on your back with your arms at your sides. **Activate your powerhouse.** Lift your legs to form a 90-degree angle—knees are directly over hips, calves parallel to the floor, toes pointed and above your knees. Elongate your neck and spine.

STEP 1

Inhale slowly and, using your powerhouse, peel your head and upper back off the mat, so that just your shoulder blades touch it. Your head is lifted, your arms are raised 6–8 inches above the mat, and your chest is soft.

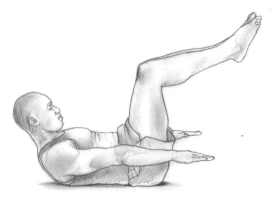

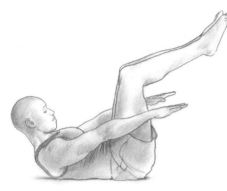

MODIFICATIONS

If this exercise proves too challenging, perform 50 arm pumps (5 full breath cycles).

If your neck tires during this exercise, rest it on the mat.

STEP 2

Exhale slowly through your nose as you vigorously pump your arms for a count of 5. Inhale slowly through your nose for 5 counts. Continue pumping your arms, inhaling and exhaling on a count of 5, until you reach 50–100 pumps (5–10 full breath cycles). Keep your eyes on your midsection as you pump. When you have completed all sets, draw your knees to your chest, lower your head, and return to the starting position. *Place your feet on the mat to prepare for The Roll Down.*

Concentration: Use your lower abdominals to support the weight of your legs. Use your upper abdominals to support the weight of your head.

Control: Keep your head and legs still as you pump your arms.

Center: Imprint your spine into the mat and maintain your scoop throughout the exercise.

Fluidity: Pump your arms with a smooth, fast, steady rhythm.

Precision: Keep your fingers long and reach them away as you pump.

Breath: Inhale and exhale on counts of 5— *inhale,* 2, 3, 4, 5, *exhale,* 2, 3, 4, 5.

CHECK YOUR FORM

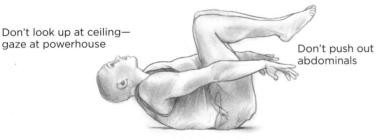

Don't look up at ceiling— gaze at powerhouse

Don't push out abdominals

Don't hunch shoulders

THE ROLL DOWN

Develops the strength to hold and maintain the scoop

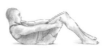

REPETITIONS
Repeat 3–6 times.

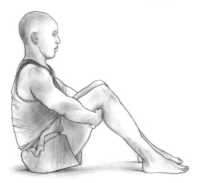

STARTING POSITION

Sit tall with your legs slightly more than hip-width apart and your feet pressed into the mat. Grasp the backs of your thighs above your knees and lift your elbows wide. **Activate your powerhouse.**

STEP 1

Contract your buttocks to grow an inch, then aim your lower back to the mat. At the same time, tuck chin to chest and look at your midsection, shaping your spine into a C-curve. Stop when your arms are straight.

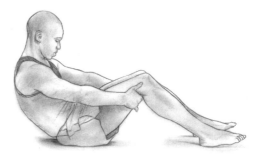

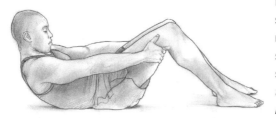

STEP 2

Deepen C-curve as you imprint your spine into the mat, opening the muscles of your lower back and scooping deeper. Curl back to the starting position. *Lower your body to the mat, arms by your sides, knees bent, for Single Leg Circles.*

Concentration: Scoop your abdominals while maintaining C-curve.

Control: Don't let your elbows fall. Keep them lifted.

Center: As you roll down, imprint your lower spine on the mat first. As you roll up, keep it on the mat last.

Fluidity: Roll down smoothly and with control. Roll back up immediately, also with control.

Precision: As you roll back up, keep your legs slightly more than hip-width apart and in proper alignment.

Breath: Inhale as you roll down. Exhale as you roll up.

CHECK YOUR FORM

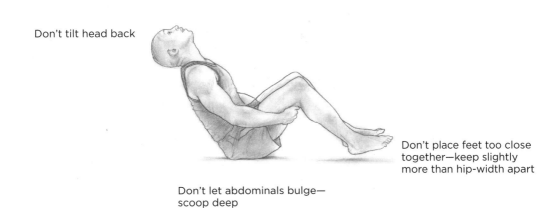

Don't tilt head back

Don't place feet too close together—keep slightly more than hip-width apart

Don't let abdominals bulge—scoop deep

SINGLE LEG CIRCLES

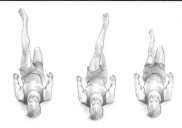

Stretches and strengthens the muscles
in the hips, thighs, and lower back •
increases flexibility

REPETITIONS

Repeat 3–5 times in each direction—clockwise
and counterclockwise—with each leg.

STARTING POSITION

Lie on your back with your arms
long by your sides and your
fingers reaching away. Rotate your
leg into Pilates stance and lift it to
the ceiling as you press your spine
into the mat. Bend your right knee
and plant your right foot on the
mat. **Activate your powerhouse.**

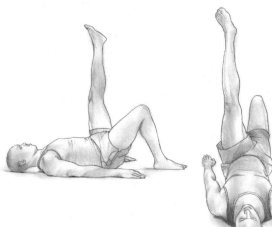

STEP 1

Inhale, then cross
your left leg up and
over your body,
toward your right
shoulder. Keep your
left hip pressed to
the mat, and work
your leg and foot
into Pilates stance.

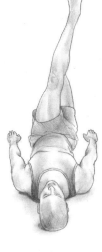

STEP 2

Circle your left leg:
Move your left leg
across your body,
then circle it down,
around, and back
up to its starting
position.

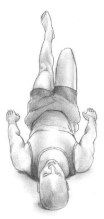

Step 3

Exhale and return your leg to the starting position. Circle 3–5 times in each direction, clockwise and counterclockwise, inhaling as you begin the circle and exhaling as you complete it. Repeat with your right leg. *Bend your knees, place your feet flat on the mat, and roll up to a sitting position. Lift your buttocks to your heels to prepare for Rolling Like a Ball.*

Modification

If you can't extend your leg to the ceiling, lower your leg to a 45-degree angle and circle from there.

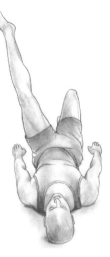

Concentration: Keep your upper body as motionless as possible. Circle from your powerhouse.

Control: Control your pelvis, circling your leg without allowing your hips to wobble. Do not allow your knee to move as you circle your leg.

Center: Maintain your scoop and contract your buttocks and the backs of your inner thighs throughout the exercise.

Fluidity: As you circle your leg, emphasize the up phase—circle *up*, circle *up*, circle *up*.

Precision: Keep your neck long.
Press the back of your head firmly to the mat to keep your shoulders down.
Pin your arms and shoulders to the mat, but keep your fingers long.

Breath: Exhale on the up phase. Inhale as you circle down.

Check Your Form

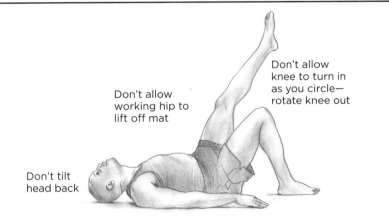

Don't allow working hip to lift off mat

Don't allow knee to turn in as you circle— rotate knee out

Don't tilt head back

Don't allow back to arch off mat

Rolling Like a Ball

Massages the back • improves balance • works the powerhouse

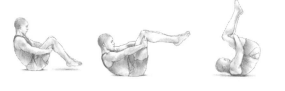

REPETITIONS
Repeat 6 times.

Caution

If you have scoliosis, omit this exercise.

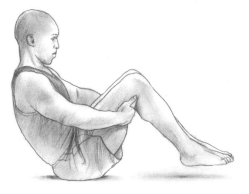

Starting Position

Sit at the front of the mat with your knees bent toward your chest and slightly open. **Activate your powerhouse.** Place a hand under each thigh (not behind your knees) and lift your feet off the mat until you are balancing on your tailbone. Tuck chin to chest and keep your elbows wide.

Step 1

Inhale and roll back onto the mat like a ball. Scoop hard and keep your elbows wide and lifted.

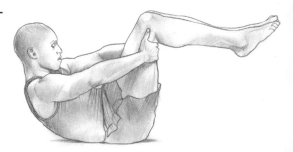

STEP 2

Continue to roll back, lifting your hips, until the base of your shoulder blades touches the mat. Keeping your ball shape, exhale and roll back up to the starting position to balance on your tailbone. Repeat. *Move back to the center of the mat and lie back for the Single Leg Stretch.*

MODIFICATION

If you can't roll, balance up with your feet 2 inches from the ground.

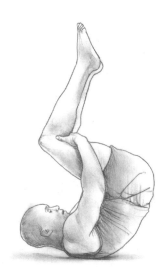

Concentration: As you roll back and forth, imagine that you are using the mat to massage your back.

Control: As you roll back, use your powerhouse to lift up your hips and balance on your shoulder blades for a split second.
As you roll down, use your powerhouse to get your lower back on the mat as quickly as you can.

Center: Maintain your scoop throughout the exercise.

Fluidity: Roll forward and back at the same speed.

Precision: Keep your ball shape throughout the exercise. To do this, keep your head as close to your knees as you can.

Breath: Inhale as you roll back. Exhale as you roll forward.

CHECK YOUR FORM

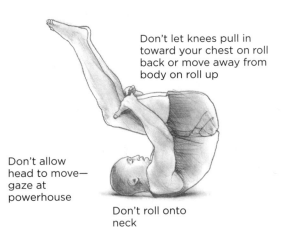

Don't let knees pull in toward your chest on roll back or move away from body on roll up

Don't allow head to move—gaze at powerhouse

Don't roll onto neck

SINGLE LEG STRETCH

Works the abdominal muscles • stretches the hips, legs, and lower back

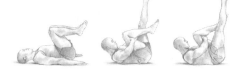

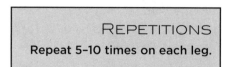
CAUTION

If your neck tires during this exercise, rest it on the mat.

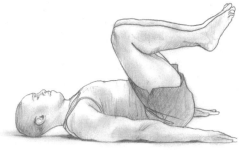

STARTING POSITION

Move to the center of the mat and lie back. Draw your knees to your chest. **Activate your powerhouse.**

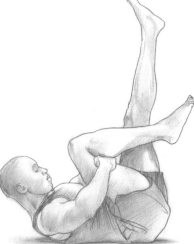

STEP 1

Lift your head and shoulders off the mat. Place both hands under the back of your right thigh, just above your right knee, one on top of the other, and extend your *left* leg to the ceiling. Keep your elbows wide as you gently draw your right knee to your shoulder.

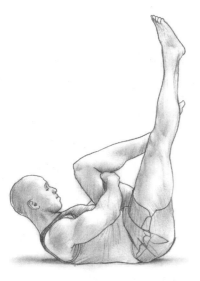

STEP 2

Switch legs: Place both hands under the back of your *left* thigh, just above your left knee, and extend your *right* leg to the ceiling. Continue to alternate legs, moving rhythmically and with control. *Hug both knees to your chest, lower your head, and grasp the backs of your thighs for the Double Leg Stretch.*

Concentration: Keep your upper body still as you switch legs.

Use your buttocks to push your foot away from you.

Use your abdominals to pull your knee in.

Control: As you hug your knee to your body, align your hip, knee, and foot.

Keep your elbows wide and lifted and your shoulders down.

Each time you switch legs, imprint your spine into the mat.

Center: Keep your Pilates box square.

Fluidity: As you switch legs, maintain a smooth rhythm. Only your legs and forearms move; your upper arms stay still.

Precision: Maintain Pilates stance as you switch legs. As your heels pass each other, they should almost but not quite touch.

Breath: Exhale when you draw your knee in. Inhale when you switch legs.

CHECK YOUR FORM

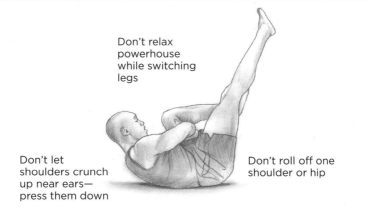

Don't relax powerhouse while switching legs

Don't let shoulders crunch up near ears— press them down

Don't roll off one shoulder or hip

DOUBLE LEG STRETCH

Works the buttocks • improves coordination • expands the breath

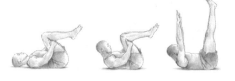

CAUTION

If your neck tires during this exercise, rest it on the mat.

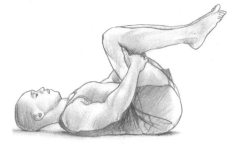

STARTING POSITION

Lie on your back with your head on the mat. Grasp the backs of your thighs, just above your knees, and draw your knees toward your chest. **Activate your powerhouse.**

STEP 1

Lift your head and shoulders off the mat, tucking chin to chest. Exhale as you draw your knees toward your chest without allowing your buttocks or lower back to leave the mat. Keep your eyes on your midsection.

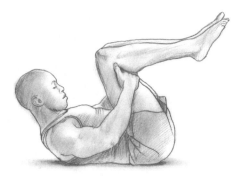

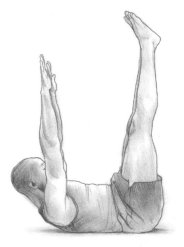

STEP 2

Inhale as you extend both legs straight up to the ceiling, working them in Pilates stance. As you extend your legs, reach your arms away from your head, keeping your arms and fingers long. Exhale, scoop, and draw your knees back to your chest. Repeat. To end, draw your knees to your chest. *Sit up tall, with your legs slightly more than hip-width apart and your knees soft, to prepare for Spine Stretch Forward.*

Concentration: Keep your head and upper body still.
Use your buttocks and inner thighs to press your feet out.
Use your abdominals to draw your knees back in.

Control: Throughout the exercise, imprint your lower spine into the mat.

Center: Work from your powerhouse: As you extend your legs, contract your buttocks and squeeze your inner thighs together.

Fluidity: Extend your arms and legs simultaneously, rather than your legs first or your arms first.

Precision: When you stretch your arms over your head, extend them straight out.
Keep your shoulders down throughout the exercise.

Breath: Inhale on the extension. Exhale on the hug.

CHECK YOUR FORM

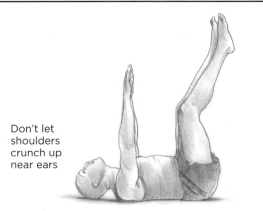

Don't let shoulders crunch up near ears

Don't arch back off mat

Spine Stretch Forward

Works the powerhouse • articulates the spine •

stretches the hamstrings

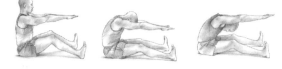

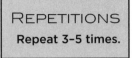

Caution

If your hips or lower back feel tight or uncomfortable as you perform this exercise, either increase the bend in your knees or limit the range of motion as you stretch forward.

Starting Position

Sit tall as though your back is against a wall. Open your legs to just wider than hip-width apart, with knees slightly bent and feet flexed. **Activate your powerhouse.** Extend your arms long at shoulder height and reach away. Squeeze your buttocks and raise up through your spine so that you feel like you've grown an inch.

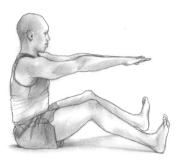

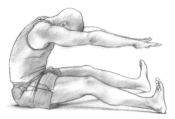

Step 1

Maintain your scoop, squeeze your buttocks to grow an inch, and start to round up and over, keeping your knees soft.

Step 2

Continue to round forward with your upper back, lowering the crown of your head straight down between your knees as you continue to reach away. When you can't roll any further, scoop your upper abdominals even more to gain that extra inch and stretch your lower back even further. Reverse the motion and return to the starting position. *This is the last exercise.*

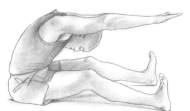

Modification

If you have a shoulder injury, place your hands, palms down, in front of you.

Concentration: Keep your hips stable as you stretch your spine.

Control: Reach in opposition. Pull your abdominals deep as you reach your body forward.

Center: Activate your powerhouse to support your lower back.

Fluidity: As you stretch, take long, rhythmic breaths through your nose. Match breath to movement.

Precision: When you reach your arms forward, scoop even harder to get that extra inch. Keep your shoulders down throughout the exercise.

Breath: As you stretch forward, exhale all your air to clean out your lungs. As you roll up, inhale deeply, filling your lungs completely.

Check Your Form

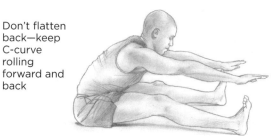

Don't flatten back—keep C-curve rolling forward and back

Don't let knees roll inward—keep buttocks activated

BEGINNER MAT

THE HUNDRED

Works the powerhouse • increases stamina

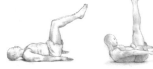 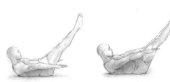

> ## REPETITIONS
> 100 arm pumps (10 full breath cycles)

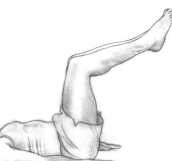

STARTING POSITION

Lie on your back with your arms at your sides; draw your knees to your chest. **Activate your powerhouse.** Elongate your neck and spine.

STEP 1

Inhale and exhale. Using your powerhouse, lift your head, stretch your arms long, and extend your legs (in Pilates stance) to the ceiling. Gazing at your midsection, pump your arms vigorously, keeping your head and upper back off the mat. Inhale slowly through your nose for a count of 5, then exhale through your nose for 5 counts. Keep your eyes on your midsection as you pump.

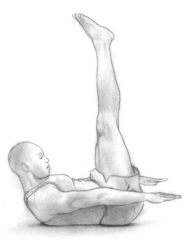

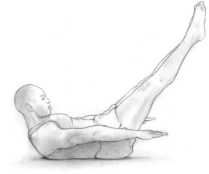

Step 2

Continue pumping your arms, inhaling and exhaling on a count of 5, until you reach 100 pumps (10 full breath cycles). When you have completed the exercise, return to the starting position. *Place your feet on the mat to transition into The Roll Up.*

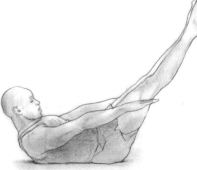

Modifications

If your back lifts off the mat as you extend your legs at a 45-degree angle, extend your legs to the ceiling instead.

If your neck tires during this exercise, rest your head on the mat.

Intermediates: For an extra challenge, lower your legs to a 45-degree angle in Step 2.

Concentration: Use your lower abdominals to support the weight of your legs. Use your upper abdominals to support the weight of your head.

Control: Keep your head and legs still as you pump your arms.

Center: Imprint your spine into the mat and maintain your scoop throughout the exercise.

Fluidity: Pump your arms with a smooth, fast, steady rhythm.

Precision: Keep your fingers long and reach them away as you pump.

Breath: Inhale and exhale on counts of 5— *inhale,* 2, 3, 4, 5, *exhale,* 2, 3, 4, 5.

Check Your Form

Don't look up at ceiling— gaze at powerhouse

Don't push out abdominals

Don't hunch shoulders

Don't lift back off mat as you extend legs

THE ROLL UP

Works the powerhouse • stretches the spine • increases flexibility

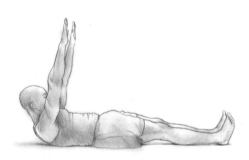

STARTING POSITION

REPETITIONS
Repeat 3–5 times.

Lie on your back with your arms stretched over your head by your ears. **Activate your powerhouse.** Extend your legs straight out in front of you; press them tightly together and flex your feet. Stretch to your full length, imprinting your entire spine into the mat.

STEP 1

Tucking chin to chest, raise your arms straight up over your head. Keep your eyes on your midsection.

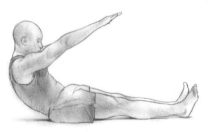

STEP 2

Inhale slowly and begin to roll up and forward, using your powerhouse to peel your head and upper back off the mat. Feel each vertebra as you lift your chest up and over your ribs, your ribs over your belly, your belly over your hips, and your hips over your thighs. Your lower back should leave the mat last.

Step 3

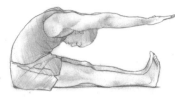

Exhale as you round over, with your spine in C-curve. Inhale as you pull your spine back down toward the mat, with your lower back touching the mat first. As you roll down, reach your fingers away, keeping them in line with your toes. When the backs of your shoulders touch the mat, reach your arms back over your head alongside your ears. Repeat. *Lower down to the mat, arms by your sides, legs straight, for Single Leg Circles.*

Modification

If you can't keep your lower back on the mat as you roll up, bend your knees slightly.

Concentration: To keep your neck long, tuck chin to chest throughout the exercise.

As you roll down and up, reach your fingers and heels away from your powerhouse.

Control: Roll up and down slowly and with control. Articulate each vertebra.

Center: Maintain your scoop and contract your buttocks and the backs of your inner thighs throughout the exercise.

Fluidity: Keep a smooth continuous rhythm. Flow through the move.

Precision: Keep your lower body as motionless as possible, and maintain Pilates stance throughout the exercise.

Breath: Inhale on the way up and exhale as you go forward. Inhale on the way back and exhale as you go down.

Check Your Form

Don't tilt head back

Don't use neck or shoulders to roll up—use powerhouse

Don't allow legs to lift off mat

Single Leg Circles

Strengthens the hips, lower back, and powerhouse •
works the outer thighs

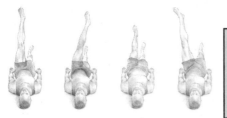

Repetitions

Circle 5 times in one direction, and
then 5 times in the opposite direction,
with each leg.

Starting Position

Lie on your back, arms long
by your sides, fingers
reaching away, with your
right leg long on the mat in
Pilates position and your foot
flexed. Reach your left leg
straight up toward the
ceiling, as close to a 90-
degree angle as you can.
Activate your powerhouse.

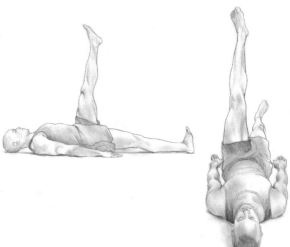

Step 1

Circle your left leg: Cross
your left leg over your
body, using your
buttocks to rotate your
leg into Pilates stance.
Maintain the rotation as
your left heel moves
toward your right
shoulder. Keep your hips
anchored to the mat.

Step 2

Circle your left
leg down and
around, toward
your right heel.
Continue to
work your left
leg in Pilates
stance.

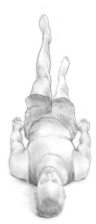

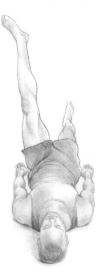

Step 3

Make a half circle, moving your left leg toward your left shoulder. Then return your left leg to the starting position. Repeat 5 times, and then 5 times in the opposite direction. Switch legs: Lower your left leg to the mat and repeat the exercise with your right leg. *Hug your knee to your chest, then rest it next to the other leg. Roll up to a sitting position and use your hands to lift your buttocks to the front of the mat to prepare for Rolling Like a Ball.*

Modification

If you lack sufficient flexibility to perform this exercise, lower your circling leg or bend your resting leg.

Concentration: Keep your upper body as motionless as possible. Circle from your powerhouse.

Control: Control your pelvis, circling your leg without allowing your hips to wobble.
As you circle, make sure your leg on the mat remains still.

Center: Maintain your scoop and contract your buttocks and the backs of your inner thighs throughout the exercise.

Fluidity: As you circle your leg, emphasize the up phase—circle up, circle up, circle up.

Precision: Keep your neck long, and press the back of your head firmly to the mat to keep your shoulders down.
Pin your arms and shoulders to the mat, but keep your fingers long.

Breath: Exhale on the up phase. Inhale as you circle down.

Check Your Form

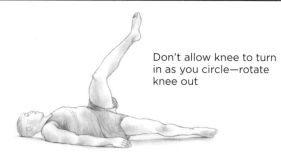

Don't allow knee to turn in as you circle—rotate knee out

Don't allow back or working hip to lift off mat

ROLLING LIKE A BALL

Works the powerhouse

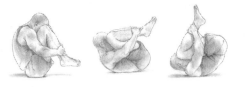

REPETITIONS

Repeat 6 times.

CAUTION

If you have scoliosis, omit this exercise.

STARTING POSITION

Sit at the front of the mat with your knees bent toward your chest and slightly open. **Activate your powerhouse.** Grasp each ankle and lift your feet off the mat until you are balancing on your tailbone and your head is between your knees. Keep your elbows wide.

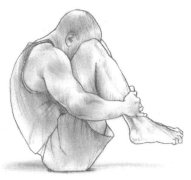

STEP 1

Inhale and roll back onto the mat like a ball. Scoop hard and keep your elbows wide and lifted.

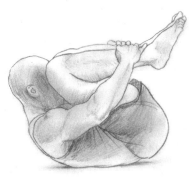

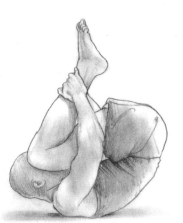

STEP 2

Continue to roll back, lifting your hips, until the base of your shoulder blades touches the mat. Maintaining your ball shape, exhale and roll back up to the starting position to balance on your tailbone. As you roll forward, try to keep your head as close to your knees as you can. Repeat. *Move back to the center of the mat and lie back for the Single Leg Stretch.*

Concentration: As you roll back and forth, imagine that you are using the mat to massage your back.

Control: As you roll back, use your powerhouse to lift up your hips and balance on your shoulder blades for a split second.
As you roll down, use your powerhouse to get your lower back on the mat as quickly as you can.

Center: Maintain your scoop throughout the exercise.

Fluidity: Roll forward and back at the same speed.

Precision: Keep your ball shape throughout the exercise. To do this, keep your head as close to your knees as you can.

Breath: Inhale as you roll back. Exhale as you roll forward.

CHECK YOUR FORM

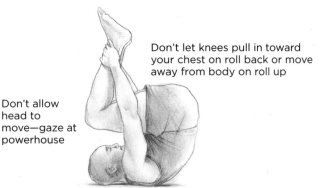

Don't let knees pull in toward your chest on roll back or move away from body on roll up

Don't allow head to move—gaze at powerhouse

Don't roll onto neck

Single Leg Stretch

Strengthens the powerhouse • stretches the hips and lower back • improves coordination

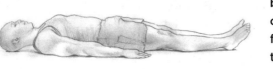

Repetitions
Repeat 5–10 times on each leg.

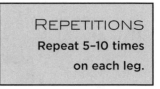

Caution

If your neck tires during this exercise, rest your head on the mat.

Starting Position

Lie on your back with your arms by your sides, your legs straight out in front of you, and your feet flexed. Imprint your spine into the mat. **Activate your powerhouse.**

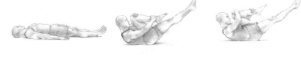

Step 1

Extend your leg. Lift your head and shoulders off the mat. Hug your right knee to your chest, right hand on right ankle, left hand on right knee. Extend your left leg at a 45-degree angle to the floor.

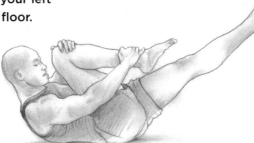

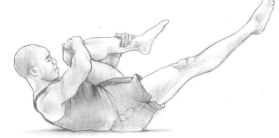

STEP 2

Switch legs: Hug your left knee to your chest (left hand on left ankle, right hand on left knee) as you extend your right leg at a 45-degree angle. Continue to alternate legs, moving rhythmically and with control. *Hug both knees to your chest, lower your head, and grasp your ankles for the Double Leg Stretch.*

Concentration: Keep your upper body still as you switch legs.
Use your buttocks to push your foot away from you.
Use your abdominals to pull your knee in.

Control: As you hug your knee to your body, align your hip, knee, and foot.
Keep your elbows wide and lifted and your shoulders down.
Each time you switch legs, imprint your spine into the mat.

Center: Keep your Pilates box square.

Fluidity: As you switch legs, maintain a smooth rhythm. Only your legs and forearms move; your upper arms stay still.

Precision: Maintain Pilates stance as you switch legs. As your heels pass each other, they should almost but not quite touch.

Breath: Exhale when you draw your knee in. Inhale when you switch legs.

CHECK YOUR FORM

Don't let shoulders crunch up near ears

Don't relax powerhouse while switching legs

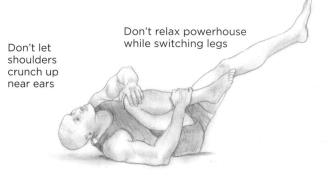

Don't roll off one shoulder or hip

DOUBLE LEG STRETCH

Lengthens and strengthens the powerhouse • stretches the entire body • enhances breathing

CAUTION

If your neck tires during this exercise, rest your head on the mat.

REPETITIONS
Perform 5–10 sets.

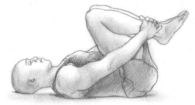

STARTING POSITION

Lie on your back with your knees pulled to your chest. Grasp your ankles. **Activate your powerhouse.**

STEP 1

Exhale and hug: Tucking chin to chest, lift your head and shoulders off the mat. Exhale as you hug your knees without allowing your buttocks or lower back to leave the mat. Keep your eyes on your powerhouse.

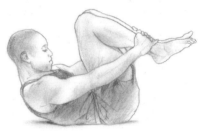

STEP 2

Inhale and extend: Breathe in and reach your arms and legs in opposite directions—arms are extended back by your ears, palms up, and legs are at a 45-degree angle in Pilates stance.

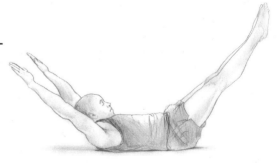

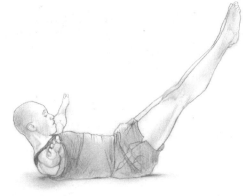

STEP 3

Exhale and return: Draw your knees back to your chest by circling your arms back to meet them. You should see both hands in your peripheral vision. Pull your knees deeply into your chest; imagine squeezing all the air out of your lungs. Repeat. *Sit up tall, with your legs slightly more than hip-width apart and your knees soft, to prepare for Spine Stretch Forward.*

For intermediate matwork, turn to page 100.

Concentration: Keep your head and upper body still.
Use your buttocks and inner thighs to press your feet out.
Use your abdominals to draw your knees back in.

Control: Throughout the exercise, imprint your lower spine into the mat.

Center: Work from your powerhouse: As you extend your legs, contract your buttocks and squeeze your inner thighs together.

Fluidity: Extend your arms and legs simultaneously, rather than your legs first or your arms first.

Precision: When you stretch your arms over your head, extend them straight out.
Keep your shoulders down throughout the exercise.

Breath: Inhale on the extension. Exhale on the hug.

CHECK YOUR FORM

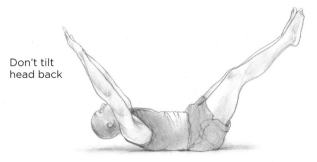

Don't tilt head back

Don't let shoulders crunch up near ears

Don't arch back off mat

SPINE STRETCH FORWARD

Lengthens the spine and the muscles of the powerhouse • stretches the back and hamstrings • enhances breathing

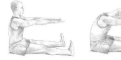 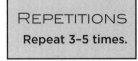

REPETITIONS
Repeat 3–5 times.

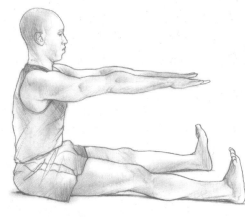

STARTING POSITION

Sit tall as though your back is against a wall, with your legs straight out in front of you. Open your legs to just wider than hip-width apart and flex your feet. **Activate your powerhouse.** Extend your arms long at shoulder height and reach them straight in front of you.

STEP 1

Maintain your scoop, squeeze your buttocks to grow an inch, and start to roll down and over.

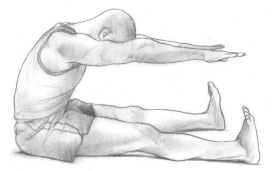

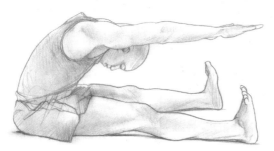

MODIFICATION

If you have shoulder problems, place your hands, palms down, in front of you.

STEP 2

Continue to round forward with your upper back, lowering the crown of your head straight down between your knees as you continue to reach away. When you can't roll any further, scoop your upper abdominals even more to gain that extra inch and stretch your lower back even further. Reverse the motion and return to the starting position. *This is the last exercise.*

Concentration: Keep your hips stable as you stretch your spine.

Control: Reach in opposition. Pull your abdominals deep as you reach your body forward.

Center: Activate your powerhouse to support your lower back.

Fluidity: As you stretch, take long, rhythmic breaths through your nose. Match breath to movement.

Precision: When you reach your arms forward, scoop even harder to get that extra inch. Keep your shoulders down throughout the exercise.

Breath: As you stretch forward, exhale all your air to clean out your lungs. As you roll up, inhale deeply, filling your lungs completely.

CHECK YOUR FORM

Don't flatten back—keep C-curve rolling forward and back

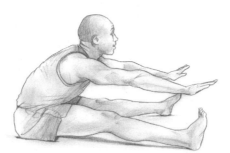

Don't let knees roll inward—keep buttocks activated

INTERMEDIATE MAT

SINGLE STRAIGHT LEG STRETCH

Works the abdominals • stretches the legs

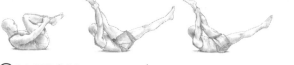

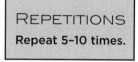

CAUTION

If you experience neck pain or strain during this exercise, rest your head on the mat.

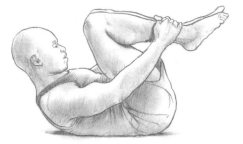

STARTING POSITION

Lie flat on the mat and hug your knees to your chest. **Activate your powerhouse.** Curl your head and shoulders up off the floor, keeping your elbows wide.

STEP 1

Turn out your right leg slightly and extend it to the ceiling. Reach up with both hands and grasp your right ankle. Exhale and extend your left leg at a 45-degree angle.

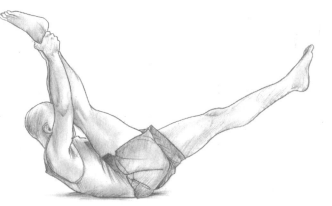

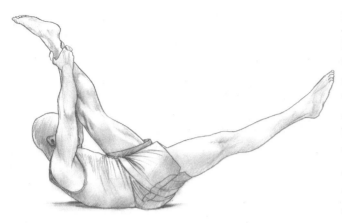

Step 2

Inhale and pull your right leg toward your head, keeping it straight. Exhale and quickly "scissor" your legs past each other. Grasp your left ankle and repeat, inhaling for one set and exhaling for the next. Repeat to finish sets. *Bring your legs up to a 90-degree angle and place both hands behind your head to prepare for the Double Straight Leg Stretch.*

Modifications

If you can't grasp your ankle, bend your knee slightly and gently hold your calf or mid-thigh.

As you grasp your ankle, gently pulse your leg twice.

Concentration: Keep your torso still as you stretch and scissor your legs.

Use your buttocks to push your leg away from you.

Use your abdominals to pull your leg in.

Control: As you grasp your ankle to your body, keep your hip, knee, and foot in a straight line. Maintain proper elbow position—raised and away from your body.

Keep your shoulders down.

Each time you switch legs, imprint your spine into the mat.

Center: Keep your Pilates box square.

Fluidity: As you switch legs, maintain a smooth rhythm. Only your legs move; your hands and arms stay still.

Precision: Maintain Pilates stance as you switch legs. As your heels pass each other, they should almost but not quite touch.

Breath: Exhale when you draw your leg in. Inhale when you switch legs.

Check Your Form

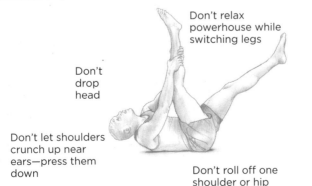

Don't relax powerhouse while switching legs

Don't drop head

Don't let shoulders crunch up near ears—press them down

Don't roll off one shoulder or hip

DOUBLE STRAIGHT LEG STRETCH

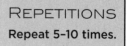

Strengthens the powerhouse •
stretches the legs

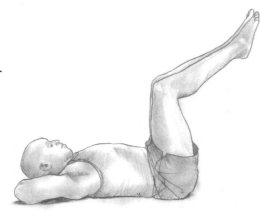

STARTING POSITION

Lie on the mat with your knees drawn in to your chest and your toes pointed to the ceiling in Pilates stance. Place your hands behind your head, one on top of the other, and keep your elbows wide. **Activate your powerhouse.**

STEP 1

Tuck chin to chest and curl your head and shoulders up off the mat, keeping your eyes on your midsection. Extend your legs into Pilates stance, maintaining your scoop.

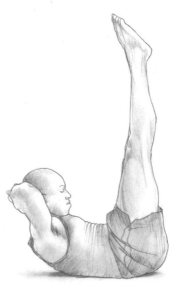

STEP 2

Inhale and slowly reach your legs away from you. Exhale and return them to the ceiling. Repeat to finish the set. *Keep your head and chest lifted and bend both knees toward your chest to prepare for the Crisscross.*

MODIFICATIONS

If this exercise hurts your neck or back, place your hands, palms down, next to your sides. You may also reduce your legs' range of motion.

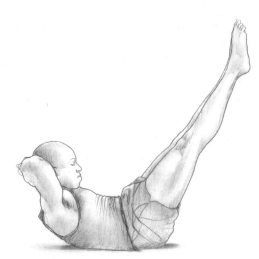

Concentration: Keep your torso still throughout the exercise.
As you lower your legs, imprint your spine on the mat.

Control: Maintain Pilates stance and scoop hard to bring your legs back up.

Center: Activate your powerhouse throughout the exercise.

Fluidity: Lower your legs slowly. Raise them quickly, but with control.

Precision: Lower your legs only to the point that your back stays on the mat.
Lengthen your lower spine throughout the exercise.

Breath: Inhale on the way down. Exhale on the way up.

CHECK YOUR FORM

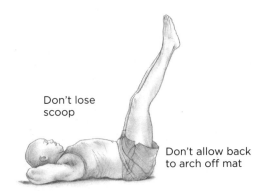

Don't lose scoop

Don't allow back to arch off mat

CRISSCROSS

Works the waistline, obliques, and powerhouse

STARTING POSITION

Lie flat on the mat and raise your head. Place your hands behind your head, one on top of the other, and keep your elbows wide. Bend your knees toward your chest. **Activate your powerhouse.**

STEP 1

Inhale and raise your torso, twist to one side, and extend your opposite leg, keeping your shoulders off the mat. Aim your front elbow for your opposite knee; your other elbow points behind you. Hold for 3 counts.

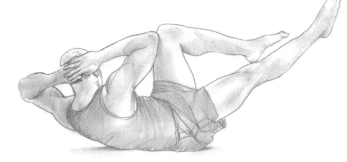

STEP 2

Exhale and switch sides; hold for 3 counts. Repeat to finish the set. *Roll up to a sitting position and straighten your legs in front of you to prepare for the Spine Stretch Forward.*

Concentration: Keep both shoulders off the mat.
Use your buttocks to push your leg away from you.
Use your abdominals to pull your leg in.
Control: Each time you switch legs, imprint your spine into the mat.
Center: To lengthen your lower back, maintain your abdominal scoop.

Fluidity: Hold for 3 counts on the twist.
Precision: As you switch legs, maintain Pilates stance. As your heels pass each other, they should almost but not quite touch.
Breath: Exhale on the hold. Inhale on the switch.

CHECK YOUR FORM

Don't pull on neck as you extend your legs—head should rest in hands

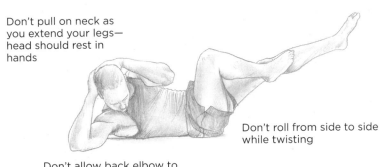

Don't roll from side to side while twisting

Don't allow back elbow to touch mat

SPINE STRETCH FORWARD

Lengthens the spine and the muscles of the powerhouse •
stretches the back and hamstrings • enhances breathing

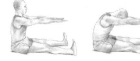 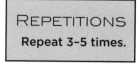

REPETITIONS
Repeat 3–5 times.

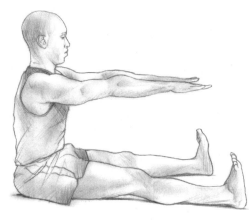

STARTING POSITION

Sit tall as though your back is
against a wall, with your legs
straight out in front of you. Open
your legs to just wider than hip-
width apart and flex your feet.
Activate your powerhouse. Extend
your arms long at shoulder height
and reach them straight in front of
you.

STEP 1

Maintain your scoop, squeeze
your buttocks to grow an inch,
and start to roll down and over.

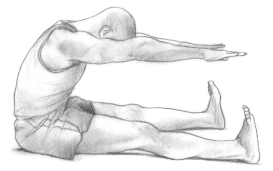

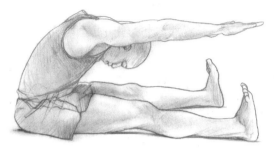

MODIFICATION

If you have shoulder problems, place your hands, palms down, in front of you.

Continue to round forward with your upper back, lowering the crown of your head straight down between your knees as you continue to reach away. When you can't roll any further, scoop your upper abdominals even more to gain that extra inch and stretch your lower back even further. Reverse the motion and return to the starting position.

Concentration: Keep your hips stable as you stretch your spine.

Control: Reach in opposition. Pull your abdominals deep as you reach your body forward.

Center: Activate your powerhouse to support your lower back.

Fluidity: As you stretch, take long, rhythmic breaths through your nose. Match breath to movement.

Precision: When you reach your arms forward, scoop even harder to get that extra inch. Keep your shoulders down throughout the exercise.

Breath: As you stretch forward, exhale all your air to clean out your lungs. As you roll up, inhale deeply, filling your lungs completely.

CHECK YOUR FORM

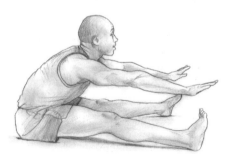

Don't flatten back—keep C-curve rolling forward and back

Don't let knees roll inward—keep buttocks activated

Open Leg Rocker

Massages the back and spine • strengthens the powerhouse • improves balance

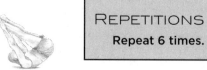

Repetitions
Repeat 6 times.

Starting Position

Sit toward the front of your mat with your knees bent in toward your chest. Open your knees to just over shoulder-width and grasp your ankles. **Activate your powerhouse.**

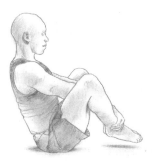

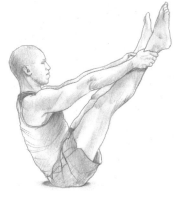

Step 1

Lean back slightly, lift your feet just off the mat, and balance on your tailbone. When you find your balance, slowly straighten your legs toward the ceiling so that they form a V. Your heels should point slightly toward each other.

Step 2

Start the roll: Inhale and roll back, making sure your back is in C-curve. Maintain your arm and hand positions—arms fully extended, hands grasping your ankles.

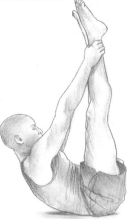

STEP 3

Stop rolling when your shoulder blades touch the mat. Exhale and reverse the roll, coming to rest once again on your tailbone. *Place your feet on the mat, then lie back, drawing your knees in toward your chest, to prepare for the Corkscrew.*

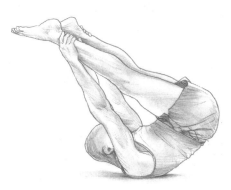

MODIFICATIONS

If you cannot fully extend your legs, keep a slight bend in your knees and place your hands on your calves rather than your ankles.

If you cannot roll back and forward, just balance in the up position.

Concentration: Use your powerhouse to keep your arms and legs straight.

Control: As you roll back, use your powerhouse to lift your hips up and balance on your shoulder blades for a split second.

As you roll down, use your powerhouse to return your lower back to the mat as quickly as you can.

Center: Scoop to maintain your balance.

Fluidity: Strive for a smooth, controlled roll.

Precision: Contract your buttocks to maintain your Pilates foot position (heels pointed slightly inward).

Breath: Inhale on the roll back, exhale on the roll up.

CHECK YOUR FORM

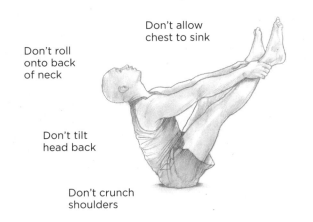

Don't roll onto back of neck

Don't allow chest to sink

Don't tilt head back

Don't crunch shoulders

CORKSCREW

Works the powerhouse • massages and strengthens the hips

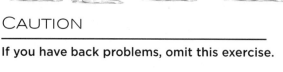

CAUTION

If you have back problems, omit this exercise.

REPETITIONS

Repeat 3 times, alternating the direction of the circle.

STARTING POSITION

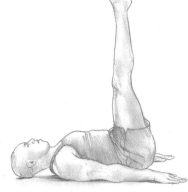

Lie flat on the mat with your legs straight up in the air in Pilates stance. Press the backs of your arms and your palms deep into the mat. Keep your neck and fingers long. **Activate your powerhouse.**

STEP 1

Inhale as you contract your inner thighs and buttocks and move your legs to your right side, keeping your heels in a V. Do not let the left side of your body lift off the mat.

STEP 2

Circle your legs down through your center line and continue to scoop your abdominals hard.

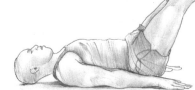

STEP 3

Sweep your legs to the left and exhale to return to the starting position. Reverse the circle. Repeat. *Bend both knees to your chest, then sit up tall to prepare for the Saw.*

MODIFICATION

If your lower back needs extra support, bend your knees as you maintain Pilates stance.

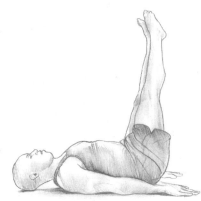

Concentration: Keep your upper body still. Only your hips and legs should move.

Control: To stabilize your torso, sink your palms into the mat.

When you circle up, don't let your feet pass your center line.

Center: Anchor your powerhouse through your lower stomach and lower back.

When you circle down, stay at the height that keeps your lower back on the mat.

Fluidity: As you circle, emphasize the up motion.

Precision: Contract your buttocks and the backs of your inner thighs to maintain Pilates stance.

Pin your shoulders to the mat to control your upper body.

Keep your chest open and your shoulders wide.

Breath: Inhale on the circle down. Exhale on the circle up.

CHECK YOUR FORM

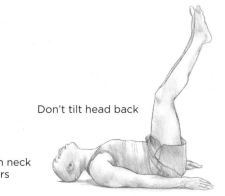

Don't tilt head back

Don't crunch neck and shoulders

Don't lift back off mat

THE SAW

Works the sides of the waist • articulates the spine • enhances breathing

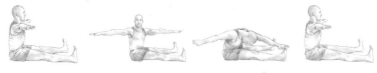

STARTING POSITION

Sit tall with your legs in front of you, slightly more than hip-width apart. Flex your feet. Reach your arms out to either side. **Activate your powerhouse.**

STEP 1

Inhale, scoop, and twist from your waist to the left. As you twist, keep your arms in a straight line and your legs and feet in position.

STEP 2

Exhale, drop your head, and round forward, aiming your little finger for the outside of your little toe. Continue to scoop your abs as you brush your little toe with your little finger. Deepen your exhale as you lift your back arm and stretch the crown of your head toward your little toe. Anchor your right hip and buttocks to the mat.

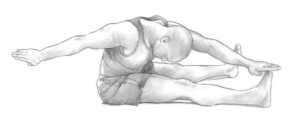

Step 3

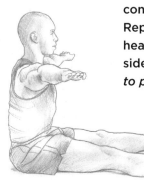

Inhale and slowly roll up, one vertebra at a time, as you contract your buttocks. Return to the starting position. Repeat: Twist from your *right* side as you stretch your head and chest toward your left leg. Repeat, alternating sides. *Bring your feet together and turn on your stomach to prepare for the Neck Roll.*

Modification

If keeping your legs straight proves too challenging, soften your knees.

Concentration: Keep your hips motionless.

Control: Keep your spine elongated as you twist.

Center: As you roll up, activate your powerhouse and squeeze your buttocks.

Fluidity: As you stretch, take long, rhythmic breaths through your nose. Match breath to movement.

Precision: Twist from your ribs while pressing your hips and buttocks firmly into the mat. Align your back arm with your front hand.

Breath: Exhale as you twist and reach forward. Inhale as you come up.

Check Your Form

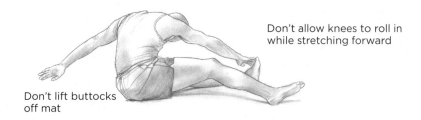

Don't allow knees to roll in while stretching forward

Don't lift buttocks off mat

NECK ROLL

Strengthens the powerhouse and back • stretches the neck • opens the back and shoulders

CAUTION

If you have back or neck problems, omit this exercise.

REPETITIONS

Perform 3 rolls in each direction—clockwise and counterclockwise.

STARTING POSITION

Lie on your stomach with your hands directly under your shoulders and your arms pressed close to your body. Press the backs of your inner thighs tightly together and place your legs in Pilates stance. **Activate your powerhouse.**

STEP 1

Lift your head and upper back, pressing your hands into the mat. Continue to arch, straightening your upper arms to 90 degrees and pressing your shoulders down and away from your ears.

STEP 2

Gently turn your head over your right shoulder and gently stretch your neck, keeping your shoulders and hips square. Continue to scoop and squeeze the backs of your inner thighs together.

STEP 3

Tuck chin to chest, lower your head, and make a slow, continuous circle, down and around to the left. Then look straight ahead.

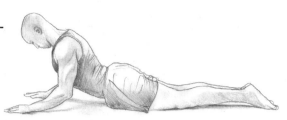

STEP 4

Gently turn your head over your left shoulder and repeat. *Support yourself on your elbows for the Single Leg Kick.*

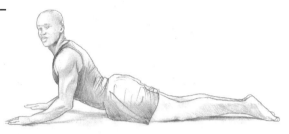

MODIFICATION

If you experience shoulder or lower-back pain during this exercise, rest your forearms on the mat with your palms flat in front of you.

Concentration: Focus your energy up and forward, leading with your chestbone.

Control: Press your shoulders down and away from your ears.

Center: Maintain the scoop in your lower abdominals to protect your lower back.

Fluidity: Circle with a smooth, continuous motion.

Precision: Squeeze your buttocks to maintain Pilates stance.

Breath: Inhale as you look to the side. Exhale down and around. Inhale as you gaze straight ahead.

CHECK YOUR FORM

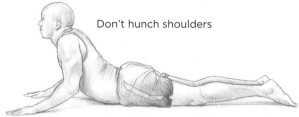

Don't hunch shoulders

Don't let abdominals go— maintain scoop

SINGLE LEG KICK

Works the powerhouse and shoulders • lengthens the back and neck • stretches the upper thighs and the sides of the hips

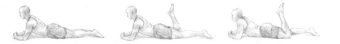

STARTING POSITION

Lie on your stomach with your forearms on the mat. Curl your hands into fists and press your knuckles together. Lift your chest. Pull your shoulders down and back and align your elbows directly beneath your shoulders. Press your thighs together in Pilates stance; touch your heels if possible. **Activate your powerhouse.** Press your hip bones firmly into the mat.

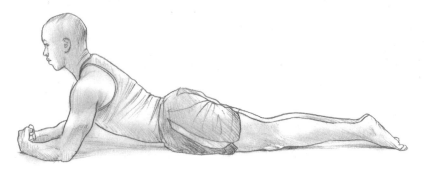

STEP 1

Lengthening your spine, quickly kick your left heel into your left buttock twice. Repeat with your right heel, kicking into your right buttock twice. Repeat, alternating legs, for 3–5 sets, inhaling for one set and exhaling for the next. *Place one ear on the mat and clasp your hands behind your back, palms up, one hand cupped inside the other, to prepare for the Double Leg Kick.*

MODIFICATION

If you find it uncomfortable to press your fists together, place your arms side by side and your palms flat on the mat.

Concentration: Lift your chest and direct your energy up and forward.

Keep your torso still as you kick your heel to your buttock.

Control: Press your elbows and fists down and into the mat.

Center: Scoop your lower abdominals to press your hipbones down and protect your lower back.

Maintain a long neck and gaze straight ahead.

Fluidity: Kick quickly into the buttock to the rhythm of a heartbeat—kick *kick,* kick *kick.*

Precision: Use your buttocks to maintain Pilates stance.

Make sure that your kicking foot and the foot on the mat are aligned with your buttocks.

Keep your upper thighs and knees together as you kick.

Breath: Exhale on the kick *kick,* inhale on the switch.

CHECK YOUR FORM

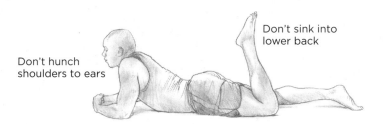

Don't hunch shoulders to ears

Don't sink into lower back

Double Leg Kick

Works the buttocks and lower abdominals • opens the
shoulders and chest • lifts the powerhouse and upper back

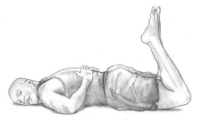

Caution

If you have neck, back, shoulder or knee problems,
omit this exercise.

Repetitions

Repeat 2 sets.

Starting Position

Lie face down with your left ear on
the mat. Clasp your hands behind
your back, palms up, one hand
cupped inside the other. Press your
shoulders down and away from the
ears. **Activate your powerhouse.**

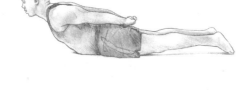

Step 1

Inhale, bend your knees, and quickly kick
both heels into your buttocks three
times. Keep your hipbones pressed
firmly to the mat.

Step 2

Exhale and, at the same time, straighten
your arms and legs, lifting your upper
body high off the mat while keeping
your hips and legs pressed firmly into
the mat. Your hands are just above (but
not touching) your buttocks. Keep your
head lifted and gaze straight ahead.

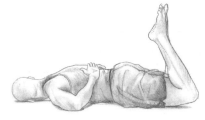

STEP 3

Lower your body, drop your head, and place your right ear on the mat. Return your hands to the starting position. Repeat. Perform 2 sets, alternating sides.

STEP 4

Sit back on your heels, head down, arms extended in front of you, hands pushing away. Try to touch your forehead to your knees to get a deep stretch in your lower back. Continue to scoop. *Roll up to a kneeling position and turn over onto your back to prepare for the Neck Pull.*

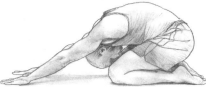

Concentration: During the reach, focus your energy up and forward, leading with your chestbone.

Control: When your ear is on the mat, your spine should make a straight line from the base of your neck to your tailbone.

Center: Keep the scoop in your lower abdominals as you kick and on the reach.
Anchor your hipbones to the mat throughout the exercise.

Fluidity: The rhythm of this exercise is one smooth, continuous motion—kick, kick, kick, *reach,* hold, 2, 3. Then, repeat with your opposite ear on the mat.

Precision: Cup your hands along your spine as high as you can as you press your elbows to the mat. Sink your hip bones and legs firmly into the mat throughout the exercise.
On the reach, maintain Pilates stance.

Breath: Inhale on the kick. Exhale as you reach.

CHECK YOUR FORM

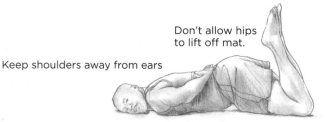

Don't allow hips to lift off mat.

Keep shoulders away from ears

Keep elbows down

Neck Pull

Strengthens the powerhouse • articulates and lengthens the spine • enhances breathing

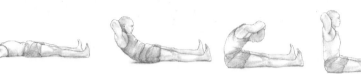

Caution

If you have neck, back, or shoulder problems, omit this exercise.

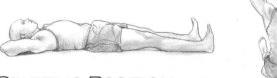

Starting Position

Lie flat on the mat. Place your hands at the base of your skull, one on top of the other. Extend your legs straight out in front of you, hip-width apart. Flex your feet and anchor your heels to the mat. **Activate your powerhouse.**

Place one hand on top of the other, as shown.

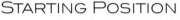
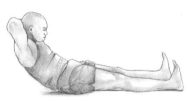

Step 1

Inhale and begin to roll up and forward, powering your movement with your buttocks. Scoop your abdominals hard and round up, peeling your head, upper back, middle back, and lower back off the mat. Roll up slowly and with control, one vertebra at a time.

Step 2

Exhale completely and round your back over your legs, pushing your heels away from your center and aiming the crown of your head between your knees. Keep your elbows lifted and C-curve in your back. Continue to scoop.

Step 3

Inhale and roll up through each vertebra to a sitting position, keeping your spine and neck long. Continue to push your heels away from your center, keep your elbows wide, and hold the base of your skull.

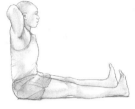

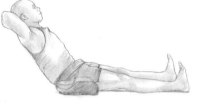

Step 4

Slowly exhale and tilt back in a flat line as you continue to activate your abdominals and buttocks. Keep your elbows wide and keep those heels pushing away.

Step 5

Continue to hinge back, pulling up on the base of your skull. (This is the neck pull. You will feel traction on your neck.) When you can't hinge back any more, roll back down to the mat vertebra by vertebra—lower back, middle back, upper back, and lastly your head—until you have returned to the starting position. Repeat this sequence 5 times. *Roll onto your side to prepare for the Side Kick.*

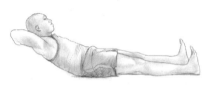

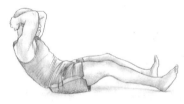

Modification

If you cannot roll up and keep your legs straight, bend your knees and wrap your arms around your head with your elbows in. Leave out the hinging motion, too—simply roll up and roll down.

Concentration: Push your heels away from your center—it will lengthen your spine as you roll up and down.

Control: Roll up and down slowly and with control. You should feel each vertebra articulate.

Center: As you roll up, keep your lower back on the mat for as long as possible.
After the hinge, as you roll down, press your lower back into the mat before your middle or upper back touches.

Fluidity: Maintain a smooth, continuous rhythm. Flow through the move.

Precision: Contract your buttocks to maintain your leg alignment (knees and toes to the ceiling) throughout the exercise.

Breath: Inhale up; exhale as you roll down. Inhale to sit up; exhale on the hinge.

Check Your Form

Don't jerk neck   Keep abdominals down

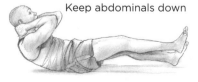

Keep legs on mat

SIDE KICK: FRONT/BACK

Strengthens the hamstrings and buttocks
Note: Perform all three Side Kick exercises to one side.
Then switch to the other leg and repeat the series.

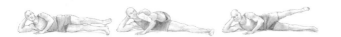

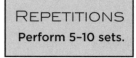

REPETITIONS
Perform 5–10 sets.

CAUTION

If you have neck or shoulder pain, perform the Modification below. If you have back or hip problems, omit it.

STARTING POSITION

Lie on your side, lining up your body against the back edge of the mat. Prop up your head with one hand and place your elbow along the back edge of the mat. Press the palm of the other hand firmly into the mat, keeping your shoulder down and away from your ear. Raise your front leg in line with your hip and rotate it slightly into Pilates stance. **Activate your powerhouse.**

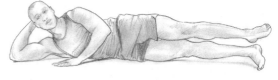

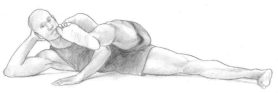

STEP 1

Exhale and use your abdominals to swing your top leg forward; pulse it twice. Keep your spine long and stack your shoulders and hips. Keep your top leg in line with your hip and parallel to the floor.

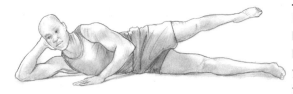

MODIFICATION

If you experience neck or shoulder pain during this exercise, straighten your supporting arm and rest your head on top of it.

Inhale and, using your buttocks, swing your top leg back, stretching the front of your hip. Repeat to complete the set, then rest your top leg on your bottom leg. *Bring your heels together and move directly to Side Kick: Up/Down.*

Concentration: Keep your top leg at hip level as you swing it forward and back.
Swing your leg only in the range that keeps your powerhouse engaged.

Control: Keep your upper body still as you perform the exercise. Move only your top leg.

Center: Use your abdominals to kick your leg forward, and your buttocks to kick it back.
Keep your shoulders back and down as you kick.

Fluidity: Kick forward and back with determination.

Precision: Use your buttocks to maintain Pilates stance throughout the exercise.
Keep your swinging leg parallel to the floor and point your heel toward the floor.

Breath: Exhale as you swing your leg forward. Inhale as you swing it back.

CHECK YOUR FORM

Don't let shoulders or hips roll forward

Don't lift leg too high

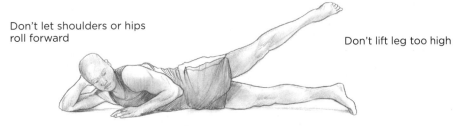

SIDE KICK: UP/DOWN

Strengthens the hips, buttocks, and outer thighs

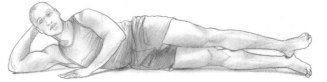

CAUTIONS

If you have neck or shoulder pain, perform the Modification on page 125. If you have back or hip problems, omit it.

STARTING POSITION

Lie on your side with your legs at a 45-degree angle, heels touching and toes forming a V. Prop up your head with one hand and place your elbow along the back edge of the mat. Press the palm of the other hand firmly into the mat, keeping your upper arm close to your body and your forearm pressed to your torso. **Activate your powerhouse.**

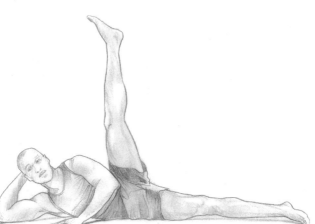

STEP 1

Rotate your top leg so that your knee and the top of your foot face the ceiling. Exhale and lift your top leg straight to the ceiling. As you kick, lengthen your spine.

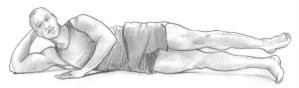

Modification

If you experience neck or shoulder pain during this exercise, straighten your supporting arm and rest your head on top of it.

Step 2

Inhale and, using your buttocks to create resistance, lower your leg. As you lower, elongate your leg so that your top heel is positioned just past your bottom heel, with your toes still pointing to the ceiling. Repeat to complete the set, then rest your top leg on your bottom leg. *Bring your heels together and move directly to Side Kick: Small Circles.*

Concentration: As you lift your leg, contract your buttocks to keep a slight turnout in your hip and thigh.

Focus on lengthening your kicking leg.

Kick your leg only in the range that keeps your powerhouse engaged.

Control: Keep your upper body still as you perform the exercise. Move only your top leg.

Keep shoulder on top of shoulder, hip on top of hip.

Center: Use your abdominals to kick your leg up, and your buttocks to bring it down.

Keep your shoulders back and down as you kick.

Fluidity: Kick your leg up with determination. Resist as you pull down.

Precision: Use your buttocks to maintain the rotation of your top leg as you kick up and resist down.

Breath: Exhale as you kick your leg up. Inhale as you resist down.

Check Your Form

Don't let hips roll back

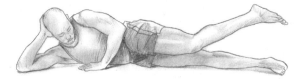

Don't let your leg rotate inward as you lift or lower it

SIDE KICK: SMALL CIRCLES

Works the hips, buttocks, and outer thighs

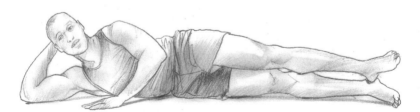

CAUTIONS

If you have neck or shoulder pain, perform the Modification on page 127. If you have back or hip problems, omit it.

REPETITIONS

Perform 5–10 circles in each direction— clockwise and counterclockwise.

STARTING POSITION

Lie on your side with your legs at a 45-degree angle, heels touching, toes forming a V. Prop up your head with one hand and place your elbow along the back edge of the mat. Press the palm of the other hand firmly into the mat, keeping your upper arm close to your body and your forearm pressed to your torso. **Activate your powerhouse.**

Step 1

Lift your top heel just above your bottom heel and circle your leg forward from your hip. Keep the circles small but vigorous, and emphasize the upswing. Circle 5–10 times, then reverse, brushing your forefoot with your top heel with each circle. *Bring your heels together to prepare for Teaser I.*

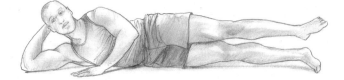

Modification

If you experience neck or shoulder pain during this exercise, straighten your supporting arm and rest your head on top of it.

Concentration: As you circle your leg, contract your buttocks to keep a slight turnout in your hip and thigh.

Focus on lengthening your circling leg.

Circle your leg only in the range that keeps your powerhouse engaged.

Control: Keep your upper body still as you perform the exercise. Move only your top leg.

Keep your thigh loose by squeezing your buttocks and softening your knee.

Keep shoulder on top of shoulder, hip on top of hip.

Center: Use your abdominals to circle your leg. Keep your shoulders back and down as you circle.

Fluidity: As you circle forward and back, emphasize the brushing of your forefoot and heel, as if you are striking a match.

Precision: Use your buttocks to maintain the rotation of your top leg as you circle forward and back.

Breath: Exhale as you brush heel to forefoot and heel to heel.

Check Your Form

Don't let hips roll back

Don't let your leg rotate inward as you lift or lower it

TEASER I

Strengthens and deepens the powerhouse • enhances balance

CAUTION

If you have neck, back, shoulder, or hip problems, omit this exercise.

STARTING POSITION

Lie on your back. **Activate your powerhouse.** Extend your legs, in Pilates stance, to a 45-degree angle. Reach your arms up and back, by your ears, with your palms to the ceiling.

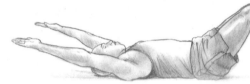

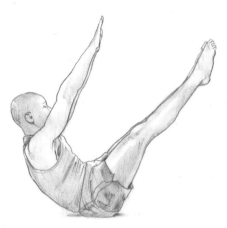

STEP 1

Lift your hands to the ceiling. Lift your head and slowly peel your body off the mat vertebra by vertebra. Reach for your toes, keeping your fingers long. Balance on your tailbone until your body resembles the letter V.

Step 2

Holding the V, exhale and begin to roll your spine back down to the mat, one vertebra at a time. When your head touches the mat, stretch your arms over your head in the starting position. Repeat twice more, inhaling as you peel your spine off the mat and exhaling as you roll back down. After the third sequence, roll to a sitting position and place your feet on the mat. *Lift your buttocks, bring them to your heels, and reach through your legs and grasp your ankles to prepare for The Seal.*

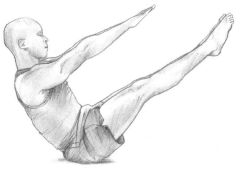

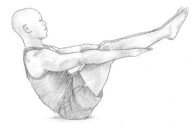

Modifications

If you cannot assume the full V, bend your knees slightly as you lift and lower your body. Or rest your heels, in Pilates stance, on a chair at a 45-degree angle.

Concentration: Keep your hips and legs as motionless as possible.

Control: Use your powerhouse rather than momentum. Do not fling up your body or flop it down.

Center: Use your upper abdominals to lift your upper body. Use your lower abdominals to hold up your legs.

Fluidity: Keep a smooth continuous rhythm. Flow through the move.

Precision: Don't lock your knees; this will tighten your thighs. To keep your thighs relaxed, contract your buttocks, which will help you activate your powerhouse.

Breath: Inhale as you lift your upper body. Exhale as you roll back down.

Check Your Form

Don't let head tilt back

Don't use hands for momentum

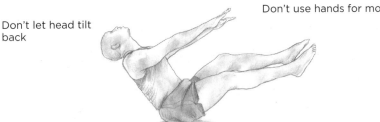

THE SEAL

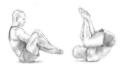

Strengthens the powerhouse • massages and stretches the back • stretches the hips

CAUTION

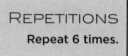

REPETITIONS
Repeat 6 times.

If you have neck, back, shoulder, hip, or knee problems, omit this exercise.

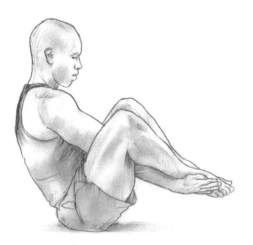

STARTING POSITION

Sit at the edge of the mat with your knees bent to your chest and the sides of your feet pressed together. **Activate your powerhouse.** Open your knees to shoulder-width and wrap your hands under and around each ankle. Lift your feet just off the mat until you are balanced on your tailbone. Find your balance.

Wrap your hands around your ankles and grasp your feet, as shown.

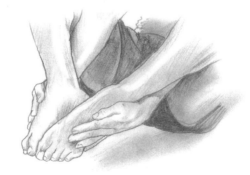

STEP 1

Inhale, roll back to your shoulder blades (you should feel each vertebra articulate as you roll back), and clap your feet together three times. Exhale as you tuck chin to chest and roll back up to the starting position. Clap your feet together three times. *Cross your legs, roll up, and stand up.*

MODIFICATION

If you can't clap your feet in the rolled-back position, clap them only on the forward position, or not at all.

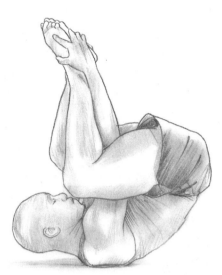

Concentration: Use your powerhouse—not momentum—to roll forward and back.

Control: Maintain your powerhouse to keep your back in a rounded position.

Center: Keep your thighs as close to your chest as possible.

Fluidity: Be mindful of the tempo of your rolling. Roll down slowly. Roll up more quickly, but with control.

Precision: Keep your feet pressed together as you roll.

Breath: Inhale as you roll back. Exhale as you roll forward.

CHECK YOUR FORM

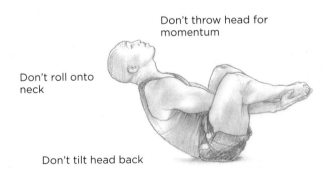

Don't throw head for momentum

Don't roll onto neck

Don't tilt head back

COOLDOWN: THE WALL

Matwork challenges the body quite a bit. This series of exercises—collectively called The Wall—helps calm it down. Performed against a wall, it helps the body transition from the mat to an upright position. The flat surface helps realign your spine, hips, and shoulders.

Note: Begin each exercise in the starting position that follows.

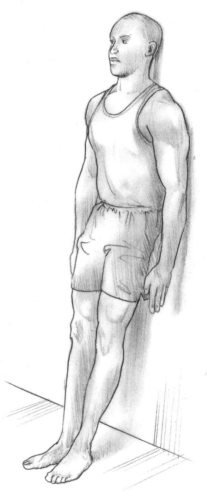

STARTING POSITION

Stand with your back against a wall. All four corners of your Pilates box should touch the wall. Assume Pilates stance. Walk out, in Pilates stance, until your lower back is imprinted against the wall. Lengthen your neck, press your shoulders down, and let your arms hang naturally. Pull your ribs in. **Activate your powerhouse.**

CHECK YOUR FORM

Don't tilt head up

Don't let ribs pop out

Don't let lower back come off wall

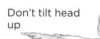

Arm Circles

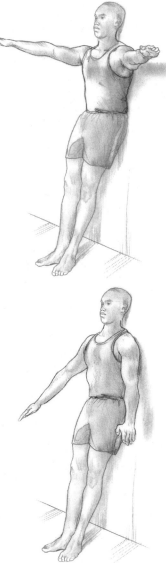

Step 1

Raise your arms to shoulder height in front of you. Continuing to press your lower back against the wall, deepen your abdominals. Keep your shoulders down and pressed against the wall.

Step 2

Open your arms, making sure that you can see them in your peripheral vision. Continue to maintain your scoop and elongate your spine.

Step 3

Press your arms down, creating your own resistance, and complete the circle with your hands in front of your thighs and fingers long and reaching away. Breathe naturally as you circle five times, from bottom to top. Reverse and circle 5 times. As you circle, maintain your scoop and keep your lower back pressed against the wall. Repeat 5 circles each way, clockwise and counterclockwise.

Check Your Form

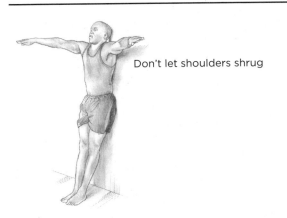

Don't let shoulders shrug

THE ROLL DOWN

CAUTION

If you have neck or shoulder pain, omit this exercise.

STEP 1

Tuck chin to chest and slowly peel your neck and spine off the wall one vertebra at a time, allowing your head and arms to hang naturally. Roll down only to the point where your lower back maintains contact with the wall.

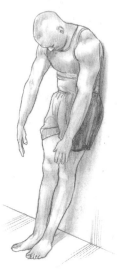

STEP 2

From this down position, make 5 small circles with your arms. Reverse, circling 5 times. Keep your arms loose and maintain your scoop. Roll up one vertebra at a time to return to the starting position.

CHECK YOUR FORM

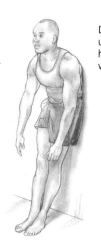

Don't roll head up too soon— head touches wall last

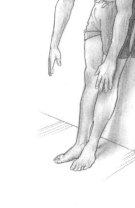

The Chair

Caution

If you have knee or hip problems, omit this exercise.

Step 1

From the starting position, stand with your feet parallel and hip-width apart, but remain against the wall.

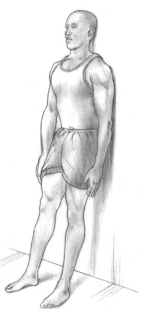

Step 2

Slide down: Bend your knees and, at the same time, raise your arms straight out in front of you, palms down, fingers reaching away. Lower your knees down until they form a 90-degree angle, with your arms parallel to the floor and even with your shoulders. Continue to activate your powerhouse to keep your spine pressed firmly into the wall. Hold for several seconds, breathing naturally.

Slide back up: Slide back up the wall, lowering your arms as you go, until you return to the starting position. Repeat 2–3 times.

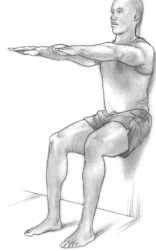

Check Your Form

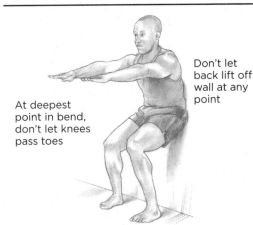

At deepest point in bend, don't let knees pass toes

Don't let back lift off wall at any point

"Chris will make you work harder on a treadmill than you've ever worked in your life. With his method, it's not enough to "get through" your cardio. You have to do it right—really concentrate on your core, posture, and movement.

Also, you sweat. This is unusual for me. The last time I worked out, a few years ago, I'd fly through 45 minutes of cardio and get a couple of beads on my lip. But Chris's method made me sweat—and I was walking at 3 miles per hour, on a very slight incline, for 20 minutes. During the press-push-pull, I could really feel the muscles in my upper body work. But because I was focusing on correct posture and movement, my glutes and my abdomen were working, too.

—*Angela*

6

CORE CONNECTION CARDIO

When my clients perform my cardio method for the first time, I never know how they'll react. Some, like Angela, rise to the challenge, exhilarated by using their minds to challenge their bodies in ways they've never imagined. Others aren't so pleased, usually because they can't read or listen to their iPods. Regardless of their first impression, however, every one of them keeps with it, because they all agree on one thing: *It works.*

If you're ready to burn more fat and calories in less time—and firm your muscles as well—you're ready for Core Connection Cardio. The routines below are the building blocks of the workouts in Part 3. They teach you to apply Core Connection Cardio principles to the machines at the gym. (If you plan to use your own cardio equipment, now is a good time to dust it off.)

Show up at your workouts empty-handed—no reading material, cell phone, or iPod. Be ready to give your all, and expect to be challenged as you retrain your body to perform an activity you may have done with your eyes closed, figuratively speaking. Just do your best and stay with it—you *are* making progress. A little Core Connection Cardio goes a long way. You use so much more of your body that even if you don't perform perfectly at first, you'll get a better workout in a third or even quarter of the time.

How hard you train always trumps how long you train. For maximum results, you want to venture out of your comfort zone to see how your body responds to just a bit more effort. For the first few weeks you may not be able to work very hard for very long. But follow my program faithfully, and before long those 10 long, hard minutes on the stepper or elliptical trainer become manageable. That's when I introduce circuit training—back-to-back bursts of cardio and strength training that ratchet up the intensity of your workout and burn serious amounts of calories.

The Press-Push-Pull technique—three simple movements that employ the inner grips, handles, or horizontal bars on cardio machines—add a unique strength component to Core Connection Cardio. I illustrate them on pages 146–147. You'll use this technique only in the Upper-Body Focus workouts in Part 3.

How Hard to Train

When fitness experts talk about the *intensity* of cardio training, they're referring to effort. With Core Connection Cardio, you train at either a low or moderate level of intensity, based on your current fitness level.

All you need to know about intensity is that when you train, I want you just outside your comfort zone. Of course, you're the best judge of that. That's why you'll use the Borg Scale, a simple self-assessment test that has you rate your level of perceived exertion.

The Borg Scale begins at 6 and ends at 20. Level 6 means no exertion at all. Level 20 means you can't work any harder. (Never attempt Level 20.

Even I don't go there.) Use the scale as you train, choosing the number that best describes your level of exertion and increasing or reducing your effort accordingly. Your rating should reflect how strenuous your workout feels as a whole. Don't focus on any one factor. Instead, gauge your *overall* perception of exertion.

If you're new to exercise, stay between Levels 12 and 14. If you've been working out for a while, you can go to Level 14, but never higher than Level 16. From time to time, try to leave your comfort zone and see how you do.

Rate yourself as honestly as you can. Remember, what feels easy or difficult to you will feel different to others.

6	No exertion at all
7	
7.5	Extremely light
8	
9	Very light. If you're healthy, this might feel like walking slowly at your pace for some minutes.
10	
11	Light
12	
13	Somewhat hard. You're working hard, but can continue.
14	
15	Hard (heavy)
16	
17	Very hard. A healthy person can continue, but really has to push.
18	
19	Extremely hard. Most people perceive Level 19 as the most strenuous physical activity they've ever experienced.
20	Maximal exertion. Don't go here, ever.

ELLIPTICAL TRAINER

When you perform the Beginner or Intermediate Upper-Body Focus in
Part 3, use the hand positions on pages 146-147.

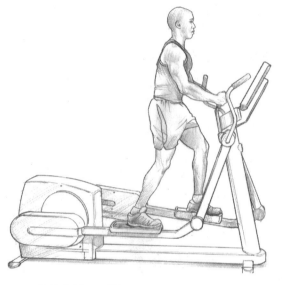

STARTING POSITION

Step onto the pedals; place your feet directly under your hips, in a slight V. Grasp the center grips (if your machine has them) rather than the bar. Lengthen your spine and reach the crown of your head to the ceiling. Get down to the core.

AS YOU PEDAL:

Keep your feet flat on the pedals—don't lift your heels.

Use your glutes to press the pedals down.

Use your abdominals to bring your knees up.

You should feel constant resistance as you push down and pull up.

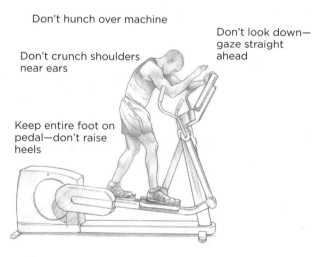

Don't hunch over machine

Don't look down—gaze straight ahead

Don't crunch shoulders near ears

Keep entire foot on pedal—don't raise heels

TREADMILL

When you perform the Beginner or Intermediate Upper-Body Focus in Part 3, use the hand positions on pages 146–147.

STARTING POSITION

Step onto the platform. Grasp the horizontal bar. As you begin to walk, imagine a straight line running down the center of the treadmill. Keep your heels on that line and your toes in a slight V. Lengthen your spine and reach the crown of your head to the ceiling. Get down to the core. Keep your body close to the horizontal bar.

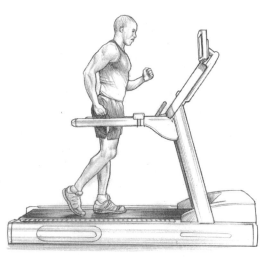

AS YOU STEP:

Step with precision. Your heels are on that imaginary line, your toes slightly off it.

Use your glutes to propel your body forward, adding power to your stride.

Point your knees straight ahead to help contract your glutes. Don't let them roll out to the side.

Step lightly—your footfall should be almost silent.

Use your abdominals to pull your legs forward.

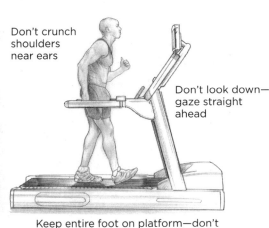

Don't hunch over machine

Don't crunch shoulders near ears

Don't look down—gaze straight ahead

Keep entire foot on platform—don't raise heels

STATIONARY BICYCLE

When you perform the Beginner or Intermediate Upper-Body Focus in Part 3, use the hand positions on pages 146–147.

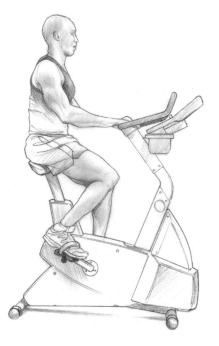

STARTING POSITION

Step onto the bike. Adjust the foot straps and fit your feet in the pedals. Grasp the handles. Lengthen your spine and reach the crown of your head to the ceiling. Get down to the core.

AS YOU PEDAL:

Use your glutes to press the pedals down.

Use your abdominals to bring your knees up.

You should feel constant resistance on push-down and pull-up.

Keep your feet flat on the pedals—don't lift your heels.

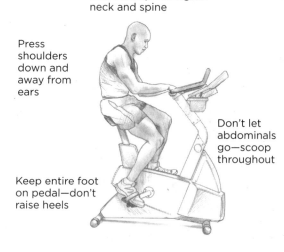

Don't slump—elongate neck and spine

Press shoulders down and away from ears

Don't let abdominals go—scoop throughout

Keep entire foot on pedal—don't raise heels

STEPPER

When you perform the Beginner or Intermediate Upper-Body Focus in Part 3, use the hand positions on pages 146–147.

STARTING POSITION

Step onto the pedals. Place your feet directly under your shoulders and place them in a slight V. Grasp the center grips, rather than the horizontal bar. Lengthen your spine and reach the crown of your head to the ceiling. Get down to the core.

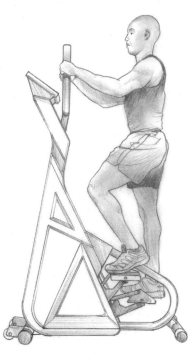

Don't raise shoulders—keep them down and back

Don't slump—stay tall

Don't relax abdominals—draw navel to spine throughout

Keep entire foot on pedal—don't raise heels

AS YOU PEDAL:

Use your glutes to press the pedals down.

Use your abdominals to bring your knees up.

You should feel constant resistance on push-down and pull-up.

Keep your feet flat on the pedals—don't lift your heels.

Outdoor Walking

After I taught my clients to use the Core Connection System on their daily walks, they were blown away by the increased level of challenge. They didn't mind—they were happy to burn more calories, strengthen their core, and protect their knees, spine, and lower back. Here's how to walk the Core Connection way.

Stand tall and activate your powerhouse. Aim the top of your head to the sky and press your shoulders down. Fix your gaze slightly downward on a distant point. Bend your elbows and hold your arms close to your sides.

As You Walk

Imagine a straight line running down the center of your path. Keep your heels on that line and your toes in a slight V.

Step with precision. Your heels are on that imaginary line, your toes slightly off it.

Swing your arms opposite your legs. As you stride, drive your elbows back and behind you, then slightly in front of your rib cage.

Use your glutes to propel your body forward, adding power to your stride.

Point your knees straight ahead to help contract your glutes. Don't let them roll out to the side.

Step lightly—your footfall should be almost silent.

Use your abdominals to pull your legs forward.

Don't pound or slap your feet on the ground. Lower your feet quietly and with control, which forces you to use your powerhouse.

Give yourself a few sessions to learn the technique. Correct and perfect as you go.

Setting the Pace

1. **Warm up.** For the first five minutes of your walk, simply amble along. This warm-up quickens the flow of blood to the muscles in your legs, prepping them for the more demanding work to come and protecting them against injury.

2. **Stretch.** Following your warm-up, perform a few quick stretches. *Toe raises:* Stand in place. Raise the toes of your left foot, keeping your heel on the ground, then lower them again. Repeat with your right foot. Perform 8–12 repetitions per foot. *Ankle rolls:* Stand in place. Lift your right foot, roll it from the ankle clockwise 8–12 repetitions, then counterclockwise 8–12 repetitions. Repeat with your left foot.

3. Once you're warmed up, begin your walk, increasing your pace steadily. At minute **8,** imagine you're walking to a meeting with your boss and you're one minute late. At minute **10,** pretend you're on your way to an IRS audit and you're five minutes late. At minute **12,** imagine you're 10 minutes late. Now *that's* walking.

4. **Cool down.** For the last five minutes of your walk, slow to a stroll. Don't skip your cool down. If you stop your walk short, the extra blood that was pumped to your legs may pool there, making you light-headed.

5. **Complete your workout.** After your walk, perform the Beginner or Intermediate Total-Body Focus in Part 3.

Press-Push-Pull Technique for Machines with Inner Grips

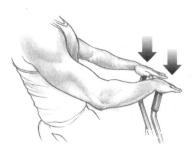

Hand Position 1: Press

From the starting position, and working from your core, press down on the bar, handle, or grip (pictured) with moderate force. Feel your abdominals deepen. Continue to contract your glutes and draw your navel in toward your spine. Imagine a pitchfork almost poking your abdomen—pull your stomach in deep; don't get stuck.

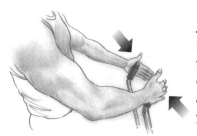

Hand Position 2: Push

From the starting position, and working from your core, place your palms on the outside of the bar, handle, or grip. Push against it, using your chest muscles. Feel your abdominals deepen as you push.

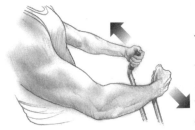

Hand Position 3: Pull

From the starting position, and working from your core, grasp both sides of the bar, handle, or grip. Pull, using the muscles of your latissimus dorsi. Feel your abdominals deepen as you pull.

Press-Push-Pull Technique for Machines with Horizontal Bars

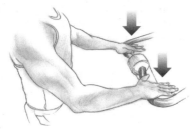

Hand Position 1: Press

From the starting position, and working from your core, press down on the bar with moderate force. Feel your abdominals deepen. Continue to contract your glutes and draw your navel in toward your spine. Imagine a pitchfork almost poking your abdomen—pull your stomach in deep; don't get stuck.

Hand Position 2: Push

From the starting position, and working from your core, place your palms on the outside of the bar. Push against it, using your chest muscles. Feel your abdominals deepen as you push.

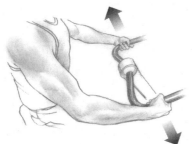

Hand Position 3: Pull

From the starting position, and working from your core, grasp both sides of the bar. Pull, using the muscles of your latissimus dorsi. Feel your abdominals deepen as you pull.

"I've lifted weights in the past, but when I worked with Chris, it felt different. Before, when I did, say, a bicep curl, I felt like I was just working one muscle—my bicep. After training with Chris, I felt all my muscles being used—my butt, my abs, my back—not just my bicep. I could really feel my core muscles working.

—Angela

7
CORE CONNECTION STRENGTH

If you fear that lifting weights will turn you into a muscle-bound Hulk, put your mind at ease: Strength training can only enhance the female body's beauty. The firm, supple muscle you build on my program will accentuate and complement your curves, but *work* for you, too.

Lifting weights builds more than muscle. It builds good health. Hang onto your muscle now, and you'll retain your independence well into old age. As a weight-bearing exercise, lifting weights improves the strength of your bones, reducing your risk of osteoporosis later in life. Studies have also found that it helps lower blood pressure and "bad" LDL cholesterol, helps raise "good" HDL cholesterol, and helps control blood sugar, which is especially crucial for people with diabetes. You'll breeze through everyday activities with more energy and a reduced risk of injury.

Lifting builds your spirits, too. Your mood brightens; your mind sharpens. You'll also burn a significant amount of calories. After a strength-training workout, your basal metabolism can stay elevated up to a day, even more than after a cardio workout. This means you'll burn more calories, more quickly, even as you sleep.

In the last chapter I showed you how to mobilize virtually all of your musculature during cardio. Now you'll do the same with weights. When you perform a bicep curl or a tricep extension, you won't just build gently rounded biceps or firm flabby upper arms. You'll firm your shoulders, back, chest, even your legs, lower back, and glutes. Remember: Train from the core, and total fitness follows.

Core Connection Strength employs just 12 exercises—six for your lower body, and six for your upper body. They're all you need to firm up fast. I provide two versions of each exercise, machine and dumbbell or body weight, for gym and home training.

If you train in a gym and haven't lifted weights before, I recommend you perform the machine versions. The machines automatically correct your posture, which reduces your risk of injury.

If you're working out at home, use the versions that employ dumbbells or body weight. I list all the gear you'll need in Chapter 3.

Core Connection Strength Do's and Don'ts

Seven years ago, before I discovered Pilates, I lifted weights with an NFL football player. We did what is called the 110 Percent Workout—find the maximum amount of weight you can lift, then lift 10 percent more than that. I was big, but I've never been so injured in my life. I was overloading my joints and giving no thought to form.

I don't lift that way anymore. I've learned that *how* you lift is as important as how *much* you lift. Whether you use dumbbells or machines, lift smoothly and with control. Don't rush, or use momentum to jerk the weight up. (If you use machines, don't let the weight stack slam the bottom plate when you lower the weight, either.) The goal is to stress your muscles, not your joints.

Keep these other points in mind, too.

■ **Activate your abdominals and glutes throughout the exercise.** I can't stress this enough. To get the most out of my method, you must consciously engage those muscles, not just the muscle being worked. As you become more familiar with my methods, it will just feel right to scoop, squeeze your glutes, lengthen your spine, and press your shoulders down.

■ **Breathe throughout the exercise.** Never hold your breath as you train with weights—your blood pressure could rise to dangerous levels. Exhale during the most strenuous phase of the movement—usually, as you lift the weight. Inhale during the less strenuous phase, usually as you return to the starting position.

■ **Lift the right amount of weight.** Lifting too little weight—or too much—compromises the effectiveness of this workout. To build strength, you must fatigue your muscles. Lift enough weight to tire your muscles after 10 to 15 repetitions. (A repetition, or rep, is one repetition of a particular exercise. A set is a group of reps.) If you struggle to get the last two or three reps in, you're lifting the correct amount. When you can crank out 12 reps relatively easily, increase the weight.

■ **Give your muscles a break.** No matter how much you want to tone your upper arms, do not train your triceps on consecutive days. You'll do nothing for your triceps but make them sore and vulnerable to injury. Always rest a day between training the same muscle or muscle group so your muscles have time to rebuild. If you are sore from a previous workout, take a day off from the weights and do a light cardio workout instead.

■ **Adjust before you sit.** Before you use a machine, "customize" it so you can perform the exercise effectively and without risk of injury. Adjust the seat for your height, and the weight stacks for the correct amount of weight.

■ **Fuel up for training.** Muscles need fuel to grow. See Chapter 4 for what to eat before a workout. Many of my clients fuel up with healthy Mini-Meals—an apple and a small handful of nuts, for example—90 minutes to two hours before they hit the weights. (For other Mini-Meals, see pages 57–59.)

■ **Get good-quality sleep.** Sleep helps your muscles recover. You can't train at your best on less than eight hours.

■ **Ask for help if you need it.** There's no need to feel intimidated. If you can't find a machine at the gym, ask. Don't hesitate to take this book with you, either—lots of people do it, and working from the book will ensure that you perform the exercises correctly. At home, if you find yourself at sea, log onto my website: www.corecoach.net.

UPPER BODY

Chest Press

Prepare

Adjust the seat so that the handles line up with your chest. Grasp the handles or inside grip. (Use the grip if your machine has one.) Sit tall and plant your feet on the floor or on the platform in Pilates stance. **Activate your core.**

Perform

1. Push the handles or grips forward until your arms are fully extended. Keep your wrists, elbows, and shoulders in line and your back firmly against the seat.
2. Return to the starting position. Repeat to complete the set.

Perfect

As you push forward, press your shoulders down.

Push through your heels to fully activate your glutes.

Contract your glutes throughout the exercise.

Maintain the alignment of your wrists, elbows, and shoulders.

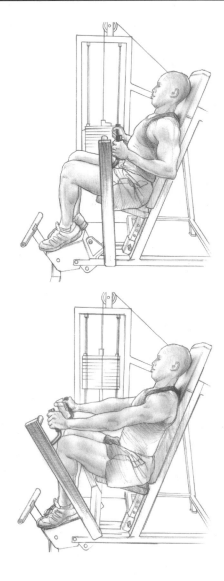

Dumbbell Chest Press

Prepare

Sit on a flat bench or on your mat. Rest the dumbbells on and above your knees. Lie back—knees bent, thighs pressed together, and feet planted on the bench or mat—and raise the dumbbells straight over your head. **Activate your core.**

SETS AND REPETITIONS

3 sets, 10–15 reps

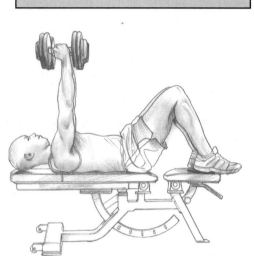

Perform

1. Contract your chest muscles and lower your arms until your elbows are at a 90-degree angle.
2. Using your chest muscles, return to the starting position. Repeat to complete the set.

Perfect

Press your lower back into the bench or mat to keep your tailbone down throughout the exercise.

Don't let the dumbbells sway back toward your head and over your face.

Really squeeze those chest muscles as you lift and lower the dumbbells.

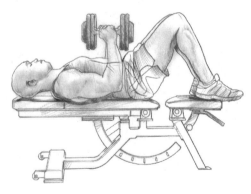

LAT PULLDOWN

PREPARE

Adjust the plates to the desired weight. Sit tall, facing the machine. Adjust the thigh pads. Stand and grasp the bar with your hands shoulder-width apart and your fingers facing you. Pull down the bar and sit, with your legs under the thighpads and your feet firmly on the floor. Lean slightly backward and extend your arms, but keep your elbows soft. **Activate your core.**

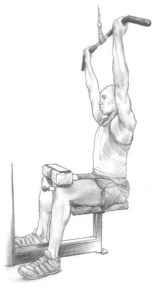

PERFORM

1. Pull the bar down until it touches your chest. Pause. Feel your abdominals deepen.
2. Return to the starting position. Repeat to complete the set.

PERFECT

As you pull the bar down, press your shoulders down.

Contract your abdominals and glutes and elongate your spine throughout the exercise.

Keep your torso still. Do not swing or lean back.

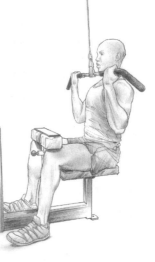

LAT PULLDOWN WITH RESISTANCE BAND

SETS AND REPETITIONS
3 sets, 10–15 reps

PREPARE

Loop one end of a resistance band around a doorknob (or use your door attachment); tug a few times to ensure that it is securely fastened. Grasp the handle of the other end in your right hand. Lie on your mat with your left arm long by your side. Reach your right hand forward so that your bicep is even with your right ear.

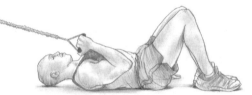

PERFORM

1. Contract your lat and pull the band to your hip bone. Feel the work in your lat.
2. Return to the starting position. Repeat to complete the set.

PERFECT

Keep both shoulders down and away from your ears.

Contract your glutes and abdominals throughout the exercise to help stabilize your body. Move only your working arm.

ROWING

PREPARE

Adjust the plates to the desired weight. Sit tall facing the machine and grasp the handles. (Use the inside grips, if available.) Place your feet on the platform, keeping a slight bend in your knees. **Activate your core.**

PERFORM

1. Pull back on the handles until your elbows are just past a 90-degree angle. Keep your neck and spine long and your elbows close to your sides. Hold for one count.
2. Return to the starting position. Repeat to complete the set.

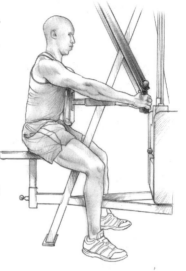

PERFECT

To elongate your spine, scoop and contract your glutes throughout the exercise.

Push through your heels to fully activate your glutes.

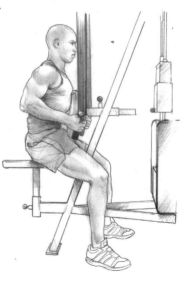

Bench One-arm Row

Sets and repetitions

3 sets, 10–15 reps

Prepare

Stand to the left of a flat bench or chair and raise your left heel slightly. Rest your right knee and right palm on the bench to support your weight. Look down at the bench or chair. Keep your back straight, like a tabletop, and align your neck and spine. **Activate your core.** Grasp a dumbbell with your left hand and allow your arm to hang down naturally, in line with your shoulder.

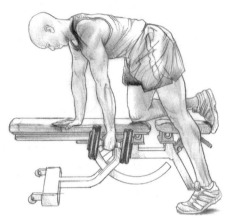

Perform

1. Pull the dumbbell up and back toward your hip, keeping your elbow close to your body. Hold for one count.
2. Return to the starting position. Repeat to complete the set, then switch arms.

Perfect

Contract your abdominals to maintain the tabletop position.

Align your head with your spine. Do not allow your head to hang.

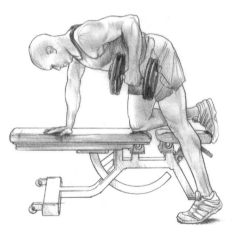

SHOULDER PRESS

PREPARE

Adjust the plates to the desired weight. Adjust the seat height so that the handles are 4 inches above your shoulders. Sit tall with your lower back against the seat, your feet flat on the floor (or on the platform, if your machine has one), and your knees at a 90-degree angle. Grasp the inside grip (if available), palms facing up, elbows at slightly less than 90 degrees. Elongate your spine and press your shoulders down. **Activate your core.**

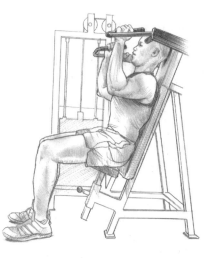

PERFORM

1. Press the handles upward until your arms are fully extended. Keep your elbows soft and aligned with your wrists.
2. Return to the starting position. Repeat to complete the set.

PERFECT

Keep your lower back against the seat.

Push through your heels to fully activate your glutes.

To elongate your spine, contract your abdominals and glutes throughout the exercise.

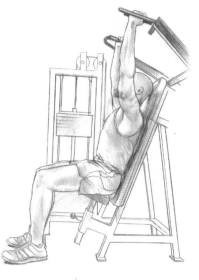

Dumbbell Shoulder Press

SETS AND REPETITIONS
3 sets, 10–15 reps

Prepare

Sit tall on a flat bench or chair with your feet flat on the floor, shoulder-width apart, in Pilates stance. **Activate your core.** Grasp the dumbbells with your palms facing each other. Lift the dumbbells to shoulder height, keeping your wrists directly over your elbows.

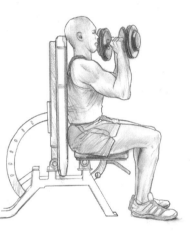

Perform

1. Slowly press the dumbbells toward the ceiling until your arms are extended over your head. Stop before your elbows lock.
2. Slowly lower the dumbbells to shoulder height. Repeat to complete the set.

Perfect

Keep your lower back against the seat throughout the exercise.

Push through your heels to fully activate your glutes.

To elongate your spine, contract your abdominals and glutes throughout the exercise.

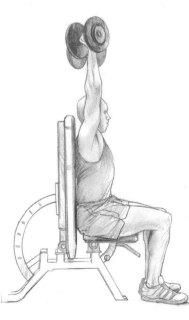

SEATED BICEPS CURL

Note: Biceps machines feature a variety of arm supports. Regardless of the type, your shoulders should always form a 90-degree angle to your hips, and your knees and hips form slightly more than a 90-degree angle.

> ## SETS AND REPETITIONS
> **3 sets, 10–15 reps**

PREPARE

Adjust the plates to the desired weight. Sit tall with your chest against the support, your entire back against the seat, and your feet flat on the floor in Pilates stance. Place your arms over the pad, palms up. Grasp the handles, keeping your arms parallel to each other. Elongate your spine and press your shoulders down. **Activate your core.**

PERFORM

1. Pull the bar up to a full range of motion. Keep your shoulders down.
2. Return slowly to the starting position. Repeat to complete the set.

PERFECT

To elongate your spine, contract your abdominals and glutes throughout the exercise.

Push through your heels to fully activate your glutes.

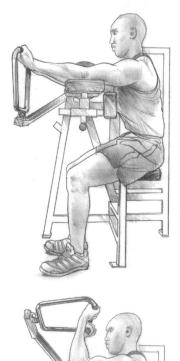

Seated Biceps Curl

SETS AND REPETITIONS

3 sets, 10–15 reps

Prepare

Sit on an angled bench adjusted to a seated position or in a straight-backed chair. Sit tall, with your back flat against the back of the bench or chair, arms at your sides, a dumbbell in each hand, palms facing forward. Elongate your spine and press your shoulders down. **Activate your core.**

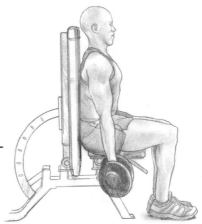

Perform

1. Lift both dumbbells toward your shoulders. Keep your elbows slightly forward and close to your body.
2. Slowly lower the dumbbells to the starting position. Repeat to complete the set.

Perfect

Keep your upper arms and torso still as you lift and lower the weights. Do not use momentum to swing the weight up.

As you lift and lower, push through your heels to fully activate your glutes.

Keep your elbows slightly forward as you lower and lift.

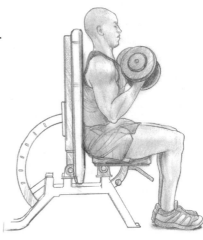

CABLE TRICEPS EXTENSION

Note: Use the angled grip to perform this exercise.

PREPARE

Adjust the plates to the desired weight. Face the machine in Pilates stance, knees soft, elbows back and close to your body. Grasp the handles in an underhand grip, palms down. **Activate your core.**

PERFORM

1. Inhale slowly, then exhale and lower the grip without moving your elbows. Contract your triceps; hold for one count. Feel your stomach deepen. Contract your glutes.
2. Return to the starting position. Repeat to complete the set.

PERFECT

Lean slightly forward. Make your body one straight line from shoulders to ankles.

Keep your elbows slightly forward throughout the exercise. Don't let them wobble forward or backward; move only your forearms.

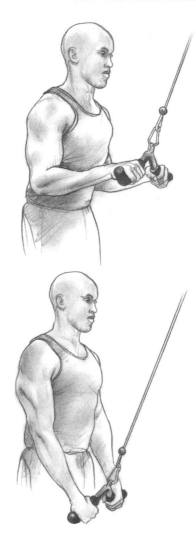

Triceps Kickback

SETS AND REPETITIONS
3 sets, 10–15 reps

Prepare

Stand to the left of a flat bench or chair and raise your left heel slightly. Rest your right knee and right palm on the bench to support your weight. Look at the floor. Keep your back straight, like a tabletop, but align your neck and spine. Grasp a dumbbell with your left hand and raise it to your hip. **Activate your core.**

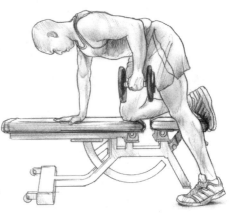

Perform

1. Keeping your back straight, pull the dumbbell straight back and up to your side until it is parallel to the floor.
2. Extend your arm until your wrist, elbow, and shoulder align.
3. Return to the starting position. Repeat to complete the set, then switch arms.

Perfect

Contract your abdominals to maintain the tabletop position.

Align your head with your spine. Do not allow your head to hang.

Keep your upper arm motionless and close to your body.

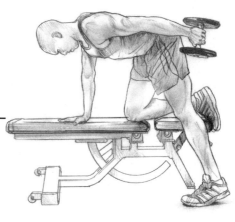

LOWER BODY

Step-back Lunge
(beginner)

Sets and repetitions
3 sets, 10–15 reps

Prepare

Stand in front of a sturdy chair and rest your palms on the top. Assume Pilates stance. Elongate your spine and reach the top of your head to the ceiling. **Activate your core.**

Perform

1. Inhale and step back: Inhale and, with control, step *back* with your left leg, pushing through your heel. Keep your knee above your ankle and drop your left knee to about 6 inches from the floor.
Note: Your right thigh is not quite parallel to the floor.
2. As you step back, lunge directly down, pressing down on the top of the chair to activate your abdominals. Keep your spine long and your head lifted.
3. Exhale and use your glutes to return to the starting position. Bring your feet together, contract your glutes, and lunge, again pressing through your heel.
4. Repeat to complete the set, then switch legs.

Perfect

Press your shoulders down throughout the exercise.

Scoop throughout the exercise to keep your upper body still and your spine long.

To stabilize your working leg, contract your glutes.

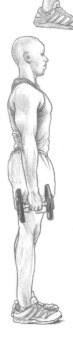

Dumbbell Step-back Lunge (intermediate)

Prepare

Hold the dumbbells at your sides, palms facing in. Assume Pilates stance. Elongate your spine and reach the top of your head to the ceiling. **Activate your core.**

Perform

1. Inhale and step back: Inhale and, with control, step *back* with your left leg, pushing through your heel. Keep your knee above your ankle and drop your left knee to about 6 inches from the floor. **Note:** Your right thigh is not quite parallel to the floor.
2. As you step back, lunge directly down. Keep your spine long and your head lifted.
3. Exhale and use your glutes to return to the starting position. Bring your feet together, contract your glutes, and lunge, again pressing through your heel.
4. Repeat to complete the set, then switch legs.

Perfect

Press your shoulders down throughout the exercise.

Don't let the dumbbells swing. Keep them still and close to your body.

Scoop throughout the exercise to keep your upper body still and your spine long.

To stabilize your working leg, contract your glutes.

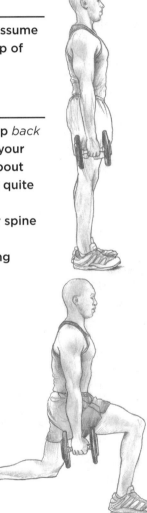

LEG EXTENSION

SETS AND REPETITIONS
3 sets, 10–15 reps

PREPARE

Adjust the plates to the desired weight. Sit tall on the machine; press your thighs together and keep your lower back against the seat. Place your shins under the shin pad so that the pad rests on your lower shins (not your ankles). Elongate your spine and press your shoulders down. Grasp the handles. **Activate your core.**

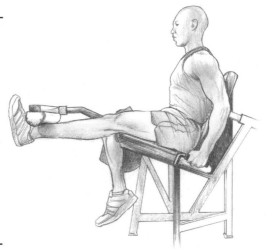

PERFORM

1. Slowly extend *only* your left leg. Stop just before your leg is straight.
2. Return to the starting position.
3. Repeat with *only* your right leg. Alternate legs to finish the set.

PERFECT

As you extend your leg, deepen your abdominals and wrap your glute, which will rotate your thigh slightly outward.

Sit tall and elongate your spine throughout the exercise.

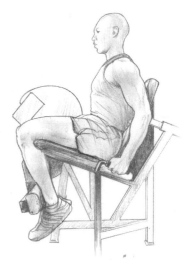

Leg Extension Using Body Weight

> ## Sets and repetitions
> 3 sets, 10–15 reps each leg

Prepare

Sit tall in a straight-backed chair with your spine and glutes against its back and your feet together and flat on the floor. Extend your arms by your sides, palms pressing away, fingers reaching toward the floor. Keep your spine and neck long and your shoulders down. **Activate your core.**

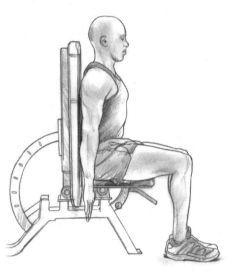

Perform

1. Slowly extend *only* your right leg. Stop just before your leg is straight.
2. Return to the starting position.
3. Repeat with *only* your left leg. Alternate legs to finish the set.

Perfect

As you extend your leg, deepen your abdominals and wrap your glute, which will rotate your thigh slightly outward.

Sit tall and elongate your spine throughout the exercise.

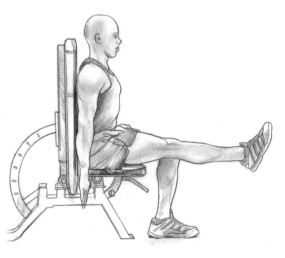

Hamstring Curl

SETS AND REPETITIONS

3 sets, 10–15 reps

PREPARE

Adjust the plates to the desired weight. Adjust the seat so that your knees clear the front edge. Sit with your entire back against the seat. Secure the pad against your thighs just above your knees. Place the back of your lower legs on top of the pad. Grasp the handles. **Activate your core.**

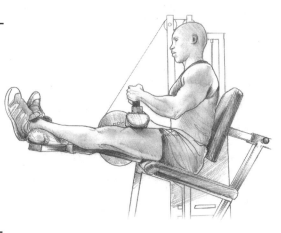

PERFORM

1. Using *one leg only*, bend your knee and push down with your lower leg until your knee forms an angle of 90 degrees or less. Pause.
2. Return to the starting position.
3. Repeat to complete the set, then switch legs.

PERFECT

Press your shoulders down and squeeze your thighs together throughout the exercise.

As you flex your leg, deepen your abdominals and wrap your glute, which will rotate your thigh slightly outward.

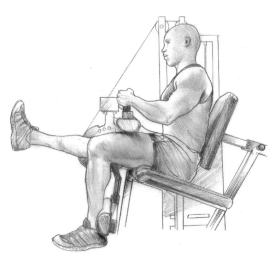

Hamstring Curl Using Body Weight

Prepare

Lean against a waist-high table, thighs together. Rest your forearms on the table, palms down; look down at the table. **Activate your core.** Align your back and head, and square your hips and shoulders. Lift your left leg straight back.

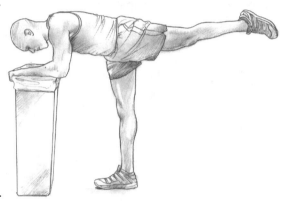

Perform

1. Raise your left foot until it forms a 90-degree angle with your knee. Contract your hamstring.
2. Return to the starting position.
3. Repeat to complete the set, then switch legs.

Perfect

As you flex your working leg, don't let your knee drop. Use your glute to keep it up.

Keep your hips still throughout the exercise.

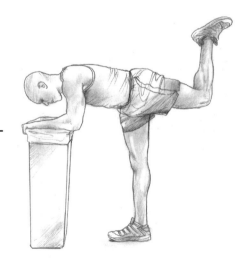

Hip Adduction

SETS AND REPETITIONS
3 sets, 10–15 reps

PREPARE

Adjust the plates to the desired weight. Sit tall with your back flat against the seat; place your feet on the bars. Pull in on the lever to position your legs wide, release the lever into position, and grasp the bars. Place the inside of your knees on the pads. *Intermediate: Do not allow your inner knees to touch the pads.* **Activate your core.**

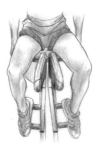

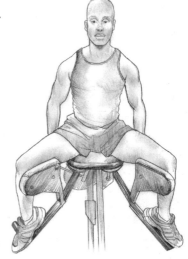

PERFORM

1. Close your legs, slowly pushing in against the resistance.
2. Return to the starting position. Do not allow the plates to touch. Repeat to complete the set.

PERFECT

Press through your heels to fully activate your glutes.

Sit tall and keep your back firmly pressed against the seat throughout the exercise.

Keep your spine long.

Don't allow your knees to roll inward.

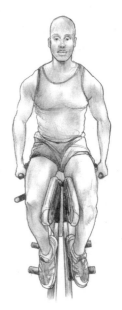

ADDUCTION USING A BALL

Note: You may use any kind of ball—a medicine ball, basketball, or soccer ball.

PREPARE

Place the ball between your thighs. Stand tall in Pilates stance. Elongate your neck and spine. Let your arms hang naturally at your sides. **Activate your core.**

PERFORM

1. Squeeze the ball between your thighs for a count of 3.
2. Return to the starting position. Repeat to complete the set.

PERFECT

Push through your heels to fully activate your glutes.

Don't let your knees roll in.

Keep your spine long throughout the exercise.

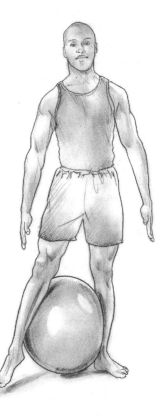

Hip Abduction

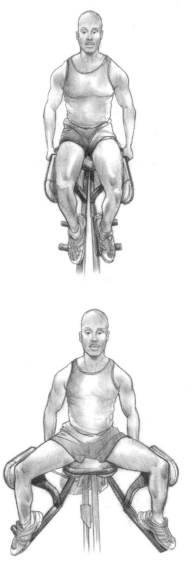

> **SETS AND REPETITIONS**
> 3 sets, 10–15 reps

PREPARE

Adjust the plates for the desired weight. Sit tall with your back flat against the seat; place your feet on the bars. Pull out on the lever to position your legs close, release the lever into position, and grasp the bars. Place the outside of your knees on the pads. *Intermediate: Do not allow your outer knees to touch the pads.* **Activate your core.**

PERFORM

1. Open your legs, slowly pushing out against the resistance.
2. Return to the starting position. Do not allow the plates to touch. Repeat to complete the set.

PERFECT

Push through your heels to fully activate your glutes.

Sit tall and keep your back firmly pressed against the seat.

Don't let your knees roll in.

Keep your spine long throughout the exercise.

Abduction Using Body Weight

> ### Sets and repetitions
> 3 sets, 10–15 reps each leg

Prepare

Lean against a waist-high table, arms straight, palms flat; look down at the table. Open your legs slightly more than hip-width apart. Square your hips and shoulders and press your shoulders down. **Activate your core.** Round your body like a lamppost.

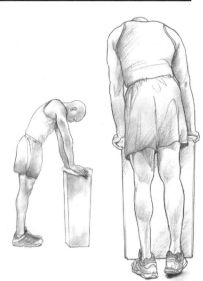

Perform

1. Place your weight on your left leg. Slowly raise your right leg, in Pilates stance, without moving your body or support leg. Keep the knee of your support leg soft, but your leg long.
2. Return to the starting position.
3. Repeat to complete the set, then switch legs.

Perfect

Press your shoulders down throughout the exercise.

Lift your leg as high as you can without leaning sideways.

As you lift your leg, rotate your knee out.

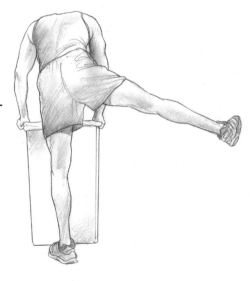

Two-legged Standing Calf Raise

Prepare

Place your shoulders under the pad and let your heels hang off the edge of the platform. Elongate your spine and keep your head and chest lifted. **Activate your core.**

Perform

1. Slowly lower your heels.
2. Stop before you reach the bottom, then push the weight back up, raising onto your toes.
3. Pause at the top. Keep a slight bend in your knees.
4. Return to the starting position. Repeat to complete the set.

Perfect

Do not allow your knees to roll inward. Rotate them slightly outward throughout the exercise.

Squeeze your thighs together throughout the exercise.

To protect your back, scoop and contract your glutes as you lower and lift.

Keep your knees soft throughout the exercise.

Standing Calf Raise
WITHOUT DUMBBELLS (BEGINNER)
OR WITH DUMBBELLS (INTERMEDIATE)

> ### SETS AND REPETITIONS
> 3 sets, 10–15 reps each leg

PREPARE

Assume Pilates stance. To increase the challenge, place your toes on the edge of a step or stair and let your heels hang off. Touch a wall for balance. **Activate your core.** *Intermediate: Follow the preceding instructions, but hold a dumbbell in your right hand, palm facing inward.*

PERFORM

1. Lower your heels to their full extent, hold for one count, then lift them as high as you can as you squeeze your calf muscles. *Intermediate: Holding the dumbbell in your left hand, flex your left leg as you lower* only *your right heel to its full extension. Then raise your right heel as high as you can, squeezing your calf muscle.*

2. Return to the starting position. Repeat to complete the set. *Intermediate: Return to the starting position. Repeat to complete the set, then switch legs. Holding the dumbbell in your right hand, flex your right leg as you lower* only *your left heel to its full extension. Then raise your left heel as high as you can, squeezing your calf muscle.*

PERFECT

Rotate your knee slightly outward throughout the exercise.

Squeeze your thighs together throughout the exercise.

To protect your back, scoop and contract your glutes as you lower and lift.

Keep your knees soft throughout the exercise.

PART THREE

8
BEGINNER:
TOTAL-BODY FOCUS

I use this workout on my clients who are new to exercise, or who have not worked out in at least one year. As a beginner, your goal is to get used to moving your body and to perform the exercises with correct form and technique. That's it, and that's plenty.

The Beginner Total-Body Focus includes:

■ Twenty minutes of cardio. As you work, stay between Levels 12–14 on the Borg Scale. Every so often, venture a bit out of your comfort zone, see how you feel, and bump up or back off as necessary.

■ A brief strength-training routine. Although it contains just six exercises, it hits every major muscle group. You will rest between sets, so you will have time to recover.

■ The Introductory mat, followed by the Cooldown. When you can perform each exercise perfectly, graduate to the Beginner mat.

To make your workouts more comfortable, efficient, and enjoyable, follow the guidelines below.

■ If any exercise proves too challenging, perform the beginner modification in its place. If the exercise does not have a modification, omit it until you gain strength and/or endurance.

■ Heed the cautions on all exercises.

■ Eat a small meal or snack 90 minutes to two hours before your workout (see pages 57–59 for ideas) and sip water throughout.

Beginner: Core Connection Cardio

Train at 65 percent of your maximum effort, using the intensity guidelines at the beginning of this chapter. You should be just outside of your comfort zone, but be able to carry on a conversation. Use correct form and technique, following the guidelines in Chapter 5. Remember, you want your powerhouse to fatigue first, before the rest of you gives out.

If you are working out at a gym: Choose two of the following machines for your cardio workout: elliptical trainer, treadmill, stationary bicycle, stepper. Work 10 minutes on each machine, following the intensity guidelines above, for a total of 20 minutes. Stop to rest if you need to.

If you are working out at home: Use the cardio machine you have. Work 20 minutes, following the intensity guidelines above. *Or* take a brisk 20-minute walk outdoors, following my walking guidelines on pages 144–145. Stop to rest if you need to.

Beginner: Core Connection Strength

Train at 60 percent of your maximum effort, tweaking the intensity of your effort as necessary. You may choose either version of each exercise, but if you're new to strength training, I recommend the machines. They place you in the correct posture automatically, and help stabilize your body so that you don't get hurt.

Perform 3 sets of 12 to 15 repetitions, and rest 45 seconds between each set. Complete each exercise before moving on to the next.

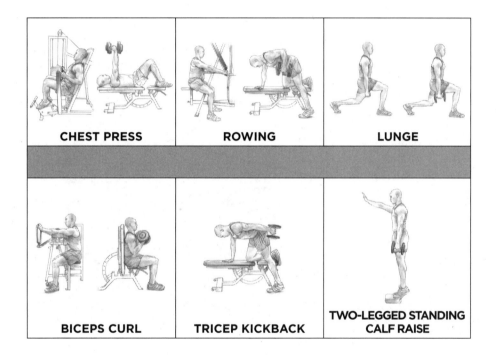

CHEST PRESS	**ROWING**	**LUNGE**
BICEPS CURL	**TRICEP KICKBACK**	**TWO-LEGGED STANDING CALF RAISE**

Beginner: Matwork

Do the Introductory mat (page 67) until you can perform each exercise perfectly. Then graduate to the Beginner mat, below. Remember your 3 C's—Concentration, Control, and Center—as well as Fluidity, Precision, and Breath.

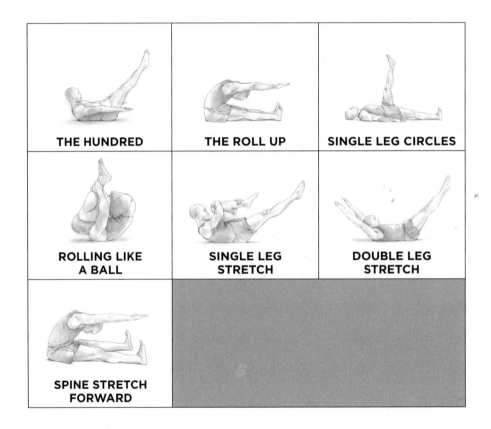

THE HUNDRED	THE ROLL UP	SINGLE LEG CIRCLES
ROLLING LIKE A BALL	SINGLE LEG STRETCH	DOUBLE LEG STRETCH
SPINE STRETCH FORWARD		

Cooldown: The Wall

Perform the Wall sequence in the order shown (pages 132–135).

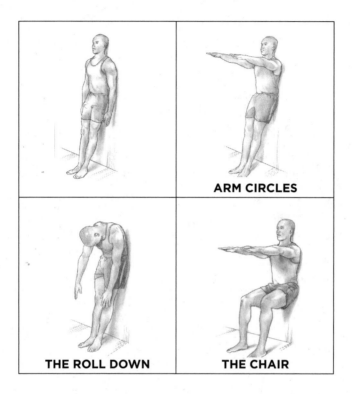

ARM CIRCLES

THE ROLL DOWN

THE CHAIR

9

INTERMEDIATE: TOTAL-BODY FOCUS

I give this slightly more challenging workout to clients who are reasonably fit or who have been working out regularly for at least six months. At the intermediate level, your goal is to continue perfecting your form and technique and building your strength, endurance, and flexibility. If you started my program as a beginner, followed it faithfully, and fueled your body appropriately, you now see a significant change in your body—less body fat, longer, leaner muscles, improved posture and flexibility. Let those changes fuel your resolve to improve, perfect, and refine your work.

The Intermediate Total-Body Focus includes:

■ Twenty minutes of cardio. Aim for Levels 14–16 on the Borg Scale if you've been working out for more than six months. Every so often, venture a bit out of your comfort zone, see how you feel, and bump up or back off as necessary.

■ A short total-body strength-training routine. You increase your maximum effort, but continue to rest between sets.

■ Pilates matwork and Cooldown. *If you have done Pilates in the past:* Start with the Intermediate mat and see how it goes. If you need a refresher, opt for the Beginner mat. *If you have never done Pilates:* Start with the Introductory mat. It may feel easy, but challenge yourself to work deep and use perfect technique.

When you can perform each exercise perfectly, progress to the Beginner mat.

When you master each Beginner exercise, graduate to the Intermediate mat.

To make your workouts more comfortable, efficient, and enjoyable, follow the guidelines below.

■ If any exercise proves too challenging, perform the beginner modification in its place. If the exercise does not have a modification, omit it until you gain strength and/or endurance.

■ Heed the cautions on all exercises.

■ Eat a small meal or snack 90 minutes to two hours before your workout (see pages 57–59 for ideas) and sip water throughout.

Intermediate: Core Connection Cardio

Train at 70 to 75 percent of your maximum effort, using the intensity guidelines on page 189–90. Push yourself a bit, but back off if you need to. Use correct form and technique, following the guidelines in Chapter 5. Remember to work from your powerhouse—it should tire before the rest of your body.

If you are working out at a gym: Choose two of the following machines for your cardio workout: treadmill, elliptical trainer, stepper, stationary bicycle. Work 10 minutes on each machine, following the intensity guidelines on page 190, for a total of 20 minutes. Stop to rest if you need to.

If you are working out at home: Work 20 minutes, following the intensity guidelines on page 190. Or take a brisk 20-minute walk outdoors, following my walking guidelines on page144–145. Stop to rest if you need to.

Intermediate: Core Connection Strength

Train at 70 to 75 percent of your maximum effort, tweaking the intensity of your effort as necessary. You may choose either version of each exercise, but I recommend the machine version and, if you're new to strength training, I recommend the machines. They place you in the correct posture automatically and help stabilize your body so that you don't get hurt.

Perform 3 sets of 12 to 15 repetitions, and rest 45 seconds between each set. Complete each exercise before moving on to the next.

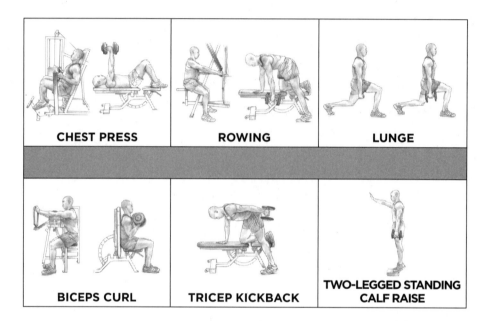

CHEST PRESS   **ROWING**   **LUNGE**

BICEPS CURL   **TRICEP KICKBACK**   **TWO-LEGGED STANDING CALF RAISE**

Intermediate: Matwork

Do the Introductory mat (page 67) and/or the Beginner mat (page 83) until you can perform each exercise perfectly. Then graduate to the Intermediate mat, below. Remember your 3 C's—Concentration, Control, and Center—as well as Fluidity, Precision, and Breath.

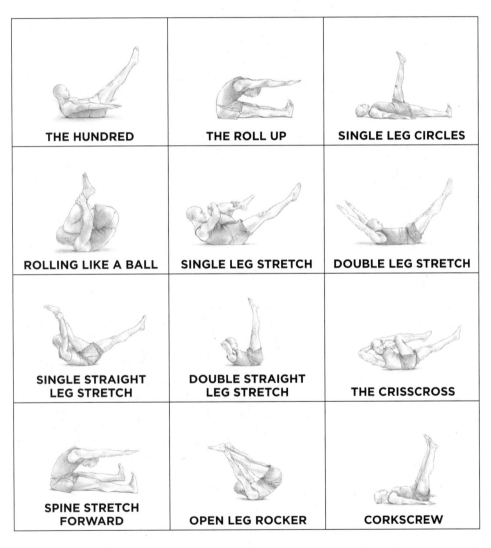

THE HUNDRED	THE ROLL UP	SINGLE LEG CIRCLES
ROLLING LIKE A BALL	SINGLE LEG STRETCH	DOUBLE LEG STRETCH
SINGLE STRAIGHT LEG STRETCH	DOUBLE STRAIGHT LEG STRETCH	THE CRISSCROSS
SPINE STRETCH FORWARD	OPEN LEG ROCKER	CORKSCREW

(continued on next page)

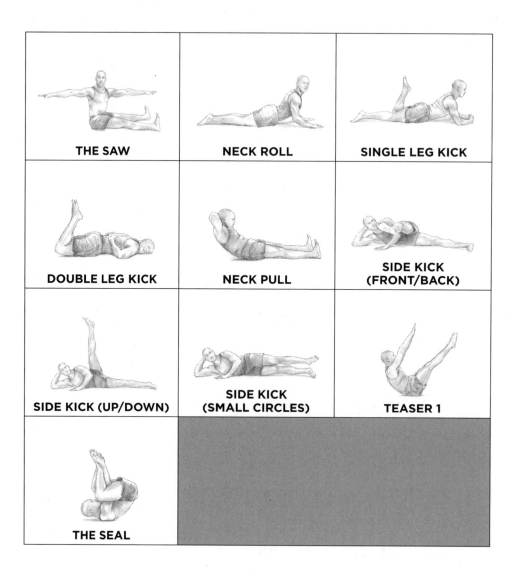

THE SAW	NECK ROLL	SINGLE LEG KICK
DOUBLE LEG KICK	NECK PULL	SIDE KICK (FRONT/BACK)
SIDE KICK (UP/DOWN)	SIDE KICK (SMALL CIRCLES)	TEASER 1
THE SEAL		

Cooldown: The Wall

Perform the Wall sequence in the order shown (pages 132–135).

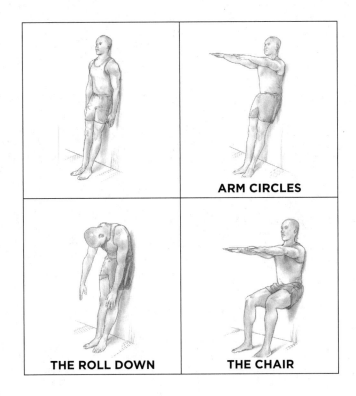

ARM CIRCLES

THE ROLL DOWN

THE CHAIR

10
BEGINNER:
LOWER-BODY FOCUS

Most of my female clients complain about their hips, thighs, and buttocks. This workout—a simple yet powerfully effective combination of cardio, strength training, and Pilates—transformed their lower bodies, and it can transform yours, too. As the cardio helps trim excess body fat, the strength training replaces flab with muscle, while the Pilates shapes and lengthens those new muscles.

The Beginner Lower-Body Focus features:

■ Twenty minutes of cardio. As you work, aim for 12–14 on the Borg scale. Every so often, venture a bit out of your comfort zone, see how you feel, and bump up or back off as necessary. Focus, too, on working from your powerhouse, working in Pilates stance, and contracting your buttocks as you train.

■ A targeted lower-body strength-training routine. Though you'll train at a higher intensity, you'll still rest between sets.

■ The Introductory Pilates mat, followed by the Cooldown. When you can perform each exercise perfectly, graduate to the Beginner mat.

To make your workouts more comfortable, efficient, and enjoyable, follow the guidelines below.

■ If any exercise proves too challenging, perform the beginner modification in its place. If the exercise does not have a modification, omit it until you gain strength and/or endurance.

■ Heed the cautions on all exercises.

■ Eat a small meal or snack 90 minutes to two hours before your workout (see pages 57–59 for ideas) and sip water throughout.

Beginner: Lower-Body Focus:
Core Connection Cardio

Train at 65 percent of your maximum effort, using the intensity guidelines on pages 197–98. Work just outside your comfort zone and pay attention to form and technique, using the guidelines in Chapter 5.

As you continue to work from your powerhouse, add a new focus: initiate the cardio movements from your buttocks. In other words, activate your powerhouse *and* contract your buttocks throughout your cardio session.

If you are working out at a gym: Choose two of the following machines for your cardio workout: treadmill, elliptical trainer, stepper, stationary bicycle. Work 10 minutes on each machine, following the intensity guidelines on page 198, for a total of 20 minutes. Stop to rest if you need to.

If you are working out at home: Use the cardio machine you have. Work 20 minutes, following the intensity guidelines on page 198. *Or* take a brisk 20-minute walk outdoors, following my walking guidelines on pages 144–145. Stop to rest if you need to.

Beginner: Lower-Body Focus:
Core Connection Strength

Train at 65 percent of your maximum effort, tweaking the intensity of your effort as necessary. You may choose either version of each exercise, but I recommend the machine version and, if you're new to strength training, I recommend the machines. They place you in the correct posture automatically and help stabilize your body so that you don't get hurt.

Perform 3 sets of 12 to 15 repetitions, and rest 45 seconds between each set. Complete each exercise before moving on to the next.

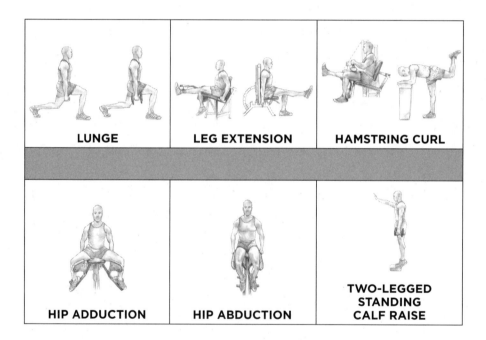

| LUNGE | LEG EXTENSION | HAMSTRING CURL |
| HIP ADDUCTION | HIP ABDUCTION | TWO-LEGGED STANDING CALF RAISE |

Beginner: Lower-Body Focus: Matwork

Do the Introductory mat (page 67) until you can perform each exercise perfectly. Then graduate to the Beginner mat, below. Remember your 3 C's—Concentration, Control, and Center—as well as Fluidity, Precision, and Breath.

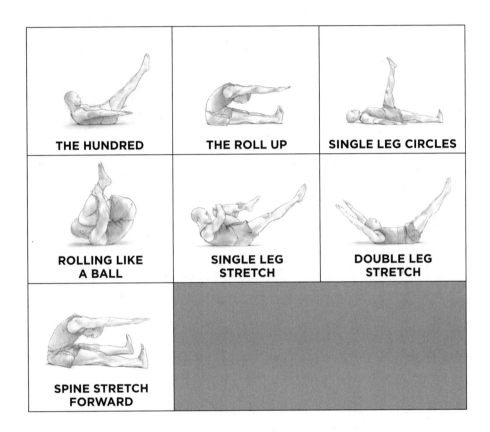

THE HUNDRED	THE ROLL UP	SINGLE LEG CIRCLES
ROLLING LIKE A BALL	SINGLE LEG STRETCH	DOUBLE LEG STRETCH
SPINE STRETCH FORWARD		

Cooldown: The Wall

Perform the Wall sequence in the order shown (pages 132–135).

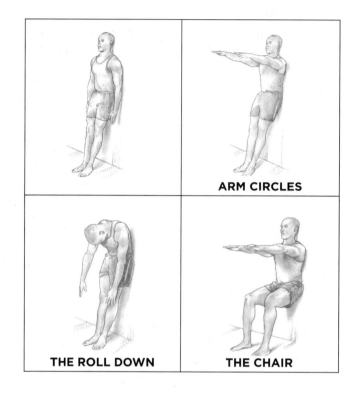

ARM CIRCLES

THE ROLL DOWN

THE CHAIR

11
INTERMEDIATE:
LOWER-BODY FOCUS

This higher-intensity program burns excess fat as it firms and reshapes your hips, thighs, and buttocks. And make no mistake: You're going to work.

The Intermediate Lower-Body Focus features:

■ A cardio/strength-training circuit, in which you alternate three short, higher-intensity bursts of cardio (24 minutes total) with a targeted lower-body strength-training routine. Aim for Levels 14–16 on the Borg Scale if you've been working out for more than six months. Every so often, venture a bit out of your comfort zone, see how you feel, and bump up or back off as necessary. Do train at the highest intensity you can—the harder you work, the more fat you'll burn.

■ Pilates matwork and Cooldown. *If you have done Pilates in the past:* Start with the Intermediate mat and see how it goes. If you need a refresher, opt for the Beginner mat. *If you have never done Pilates:* Start with the Introductory mat. It may feel easy, but challenge yourself to work deep and use perfect technique. When you can perform each exercise perfectly, progress to the Beginner mat. When you master each Beginner exercise, graduate to the Intermediate mat.

To make your workouts more comfortable, efficient, and enjoyable, follow the guidelines below.

■ If any exercise proves too challenging, perform the beginner modification in its place. If the exercise does not have a modification, omit it until you gain strength and/or endurance.

■ Heed the cautions on all exercises.

■ Eat a small meal or snack 90 minutes to two hours before your workout (see pages 57–59 for ideas) and sip water throughout.

Intermediate: Lower-Body Focus: Core Connection Cardio and Strength Circuit

This workout alternates three cardio circuits (two 10-minute circuits, one 4-minute circuit) with three strength-training circuits. You will move from cardio machine to strength-training exercise with no rest in between.

For the cardio circuits

■ Train at 75 percent of your maximum effort, using the intensity guidelines on pages 203–4. Pay attention to form and technique, using the guidelines in Chapter 5. As in the beginner lower-body focus workout, activate your powerhouse *and* contract your buttocks.

■ *If you are working out at a gym:* Choose three of the following machines for your cardio workout: elliptical trainer, treadmill, stationary bicycle, stepper. Stop to rest if you need to.

■ *If you are working out at home:* Use the cardio machine you have and train for 20 minutes without a break. *Or* walk briskly outdoors for the cardio circuits, following my walking guidelines on pages 144–145. Stop to rest if you need to.

For the strength circuits

Perform the following exercises:

■ Lunges

■ Leg Extensions

■ Hamstring Curls

- Hip Adductions

- Hip Abductions

- Calf Raises

Follow the instructions on sets, repetitions, and intensity below.

- You may choose either version of each exercise, but if you're new to strength-training, I recommend the machines. They place you in the correct posture automatically, and help stabilize your body so that you don't get hurt.

- In each of the three strength circuits, alternate sets of each exercise until you have completed all exercises and sets.

Cardio Circuit 1

Train 10 minutes on the cardio machine of your choice, following the intensity guidelines above. Follow the guidelines for that machine (see Chapter 6, pages 140–43).

Strength Circuit 1

Perform 3 sets of 12 to 15 repetitions at 75 percent of your maximum effort, tweaking the intensity of your effort as necessary. Do not rest between sets.

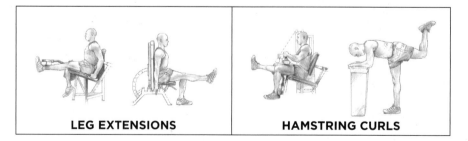

| LEG EXTENSIONS | HAMSTRING CURLS |

Cardio Circuit 2

Repeat Cardio 1. If you are working out at a gym, switch to a different machine. Follow the guidelines for that machine (see Chapter 6, pages 140–43).

Strength Circuit 2

Perform 3 sets of 12 to 15 repetitions at 75 percent of your maximum effort, tweaking the intensity of your effort as necessary. Do not rest between sets.

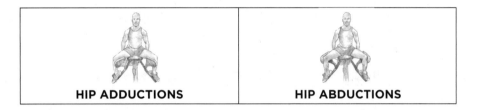

| HIP ADDUCTIONS | HIP ABDUCTIONS |

Cardio Circuit 3

Repeat Cardio 1, but for four minutes only. If you are working out at a gym, use a different machine. Follow the guidelines for that machine (see Chapter 6, pages 140–43).

Strength Circuit 3

Perform 3 sets of 12 to 15 repetitions at 75 percent of your maximum effort, tweaking the intensity of your effort as necessary. Do not rest between sets.

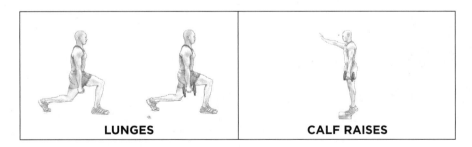

| LUNGES | CALF RAISES |

Intermediate: Lower-Body Focus: Matwork

Do the Introductory mat (page 67) and/or the Beginner mat (page 83) until you can perform each exercise perfectly. Then graduate to the Intermediate mat, below. Remember your 3 C's—Concentration, Control, and Center—as well as Fluidity, Precision, and Breath.

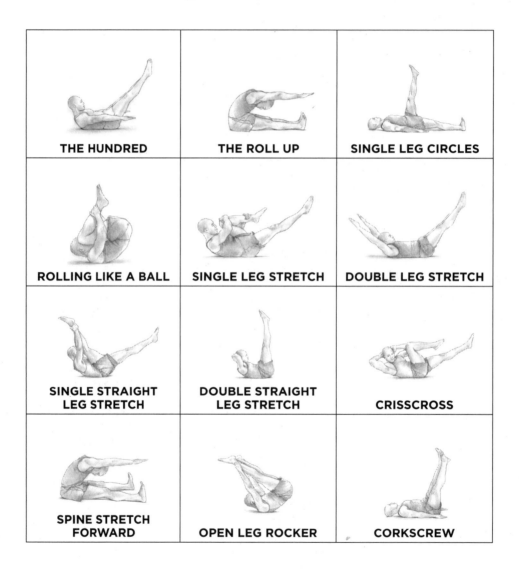

THE HUNDRED	THE ROLL UP	SINGLE LEG CIRCLES
ROLLING LIKE A BALL	SINGLE LEG STRETCH	DOUBLE LEG STRETCH
SINGLE STRAIGHT LEG STRETCH	DOUBLE STRAIGHT LEG STRETCH	CRISSCROSS
SPINE STRETCH FORWARD	OPEN LEG ROCKER	CORKSCREW

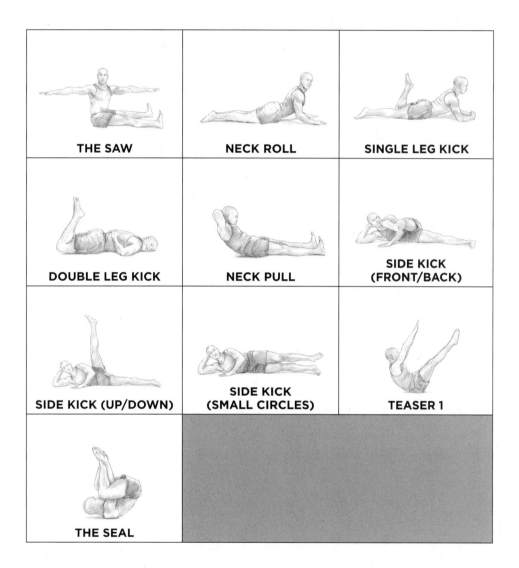

THE SAW	NECK ROLL	SINGLE LEG KICK
DOUBLE LEG KICK	NECK PULL	SIDE KICK (FRONT/BACK)
SIDE KICK (UP/DOWN)	SIDE KICK (SMALL CIRCLES)	TEASER 1
THE SEAL		

Cooldown: The Wall

Perform the Wall sequence in the order shown (see pages 132–135).

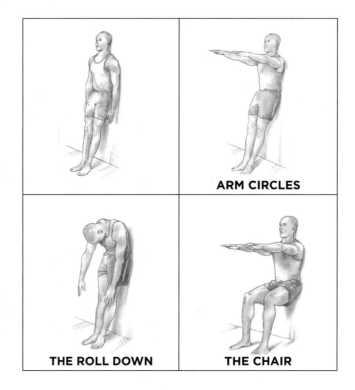

ARM CIRCLES

THE ROLL DOWN

THE CHAIR

12
BEGINNER:
UPPER-BODY FOCUS

This routine blasts fat as it firms and shapes the upper body. For the first time, you will add the press-push-pull guidelines in Chapter 5 to your cardio workout, further raising its intensity.

The Beginner Upper-Body Focus features:

■ Twenty minutes of higher-intensity cardio, broken into two 10-minute sessions. Aim for Levels 14–16 on the Borg Scale if you've been working out for more than six months. Every so often, venture a bit out of your comfort zone, see how you feel, and bump up or back off as necessary.

■ A targeted upper-body strength-training routine. You'll work at a higher intensity but rest between sets.

■ The Introductory mat, followed by the Cooldown. When you can perform each exercise perfectly, graduate to the Beginner mat.

To make your workouts more comfortable, efficient, and enjoyable, follow the guidelines below.

■ If any exercise proves too challenging, perform the beginner modification in its place. If the exercise does not have a modification, omit it until you gain strength and/or endurance.

■ Heed the cautions on all exercises.

■ Eat a small meal or snack 90 minutes to two hours before your workout (see pages 57–59 for ideas) and sip water throughout.

Beginner: Upper-Body Focus:
Core Connection Cardio

Train at 75 percent of your maximum effort, using the intensity guidelines at the beginning of chapter 6 and the press-push-pull guidelines on pages 146–47. Activate your powerhouse and contract your buttocks throughout the session. Continue to test your comfort zone, and to pay attention to form and technique, using the guidelines in Chapter 5.

If you are working out at a gym: Choose two of the following machines for your cardio workout: elliptical trainer, treadmill, stationary bicycle, stepper. Follow the routine below twice—10 minutes on each machine—for a total of 20 minutes. Stop to rest if you need to.

If you are working out at home: Use the cardio machine you have and train for 20 minutes without a break. Or take a brisk 20-minute walk outdoors, following my walking guidelines on pages 144–145. Stop to rest if you need to.

Cardio Session 1

Minutes 1-2: Using the cardio machine of your choice, press down on the handles, bars, or grips.

Minute 3: Push in, squeezing your chest muscles.

Minute 4: Pull out, contracting your lat muscles.

Minutes 5-6: Press down, as in Minutes 1–2.

Minute 7: Push in, as in Minute 3.

Minute 8: Pull out, as in Minute 4.

Minutes 9-10: Press down, as in Minutes 1–2.

Cardio Session 2

Repeat Cardio Session 1.

Beginner: Upper-Body Focus: Core Connection Strength

Train at 60 percent of your maximum effort, tweaking the intensity of your effort as necessary. You may choose either version of each exercise, but I recommend the machine version and, if you're new to strength training, I recommend the machines. They place you in the correct posture automatically and help stabilize your body so that you don't get hurt.

Perform 3 sets of 12 to 15 repetitions, and rest 45 seconds between each set. Complete each exercise before moving on to the next.

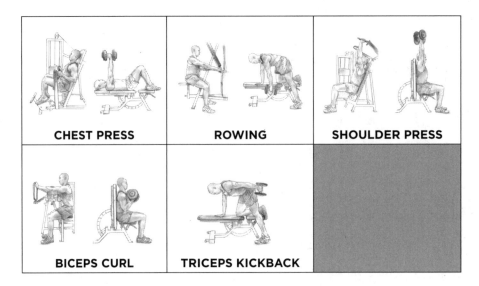

| CHEST PRESS | ROWING | SHOULDER PRESS |
| BICEPS CURL | TRICEPS KICKBACK | |

Beginner: Upper-Body Focus: Matwork

Do the Introductory Pilates mat (page 67) until you can perform each exercise perfectly. Then graduate to the Beginner mat, below. Remember your 3 C's—Concentration, Control, and Center—as well as Fluidity, Precision, and Breath.

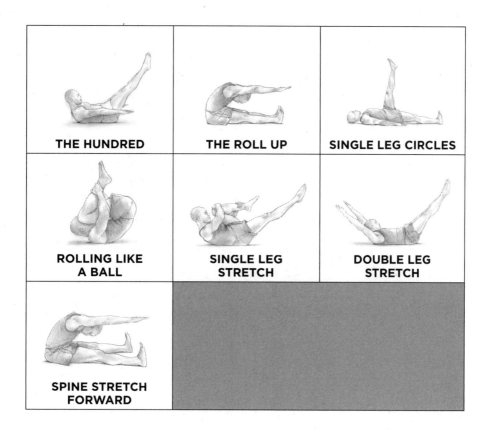

THE HUNDRED	**THE ROLL UP**	**SINGLE LEG CIRCLES**
ROLLING LIKE A BALL	**SINGLE LEG STRETCH**	**DOUBLE LEG STRETCH**
SPINE STRETCH FORWARD		

Cooldown: The Wall

Perform the Wall sequence in the order shown (see pages 132-135).

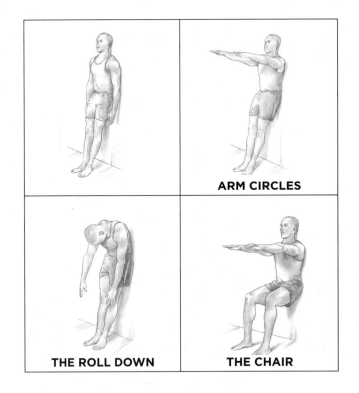

ARM CIRCLES

THE ROLL DOWN

THE CHAIR

13

INTERMEDIATE: UPPER-BODY FOCUS

In this last and most challenging routine, you'll perform a cardio/strength circuit designed to build upper-body strength. Its double dose of upper-body work burns a significant amount of calories, which will help trim excess body fat, including on the chest, back, and arms.

The Intermediate Upper-Body Focus features:

■ A cardio/strength-training circuit which alternates four short, higher-intensity bursts of cardio (15 minutes total) with three targeted upper-body strength-training circuits. Aim for Levels 14–16 on the Borg Scale if you've been working out for more than six months. Every so often, venture a bit out of your comfort zone, see how you feel, and bump up or back off as necessary.

■ Pilates matwork and Cooldown. *If you have done Pilates in the past:* Start with the Intermediate mat and see how it goes. If you need a refresher, opt for the Beginner mat. *If you have never done Pilates:* Start with the Introductory mat. It may feel easy, but challenge yourself to work deep and use perfect technique. When you can perform each exercise perfectly, progress to the Beginner mat.

When you master each Beginner exercise, graduate to the Intermediate mat.

To make your workouts more comfortable, efficient, and enjoyable, follow the guidelines below.

■ If any exercise proves too challenging, perform the beginner modification in its place. If the exercise does not have a modification, omit it until you gain strength and/or endurance.

■ Heed the cautions on all exercises.

■ Eat a small meal or snack 90 minutes to two hours before your workout (see pages 57–59 for ideas) and sip water throughout.

Intermediate: Upper-body Focus: Core Connection Cardio and Strength Circuit

This workout alternates four cardio circuits (one 6-minute circuit, three 3-minute circuits) with three strength-training circuits. You will move from cardio machine to strength-training exercise with no rest in between.

For the cardio circuits

■ Train at 75 percent of your maximum effort, using the intensity guidelines on page 217–18 and the press-push-pull guidelines on pages 146–47. Activate your powerhouse and contract your buttocks throughout the session. Continue to test your comfort zone and pay attention to form and technique, using the guidelines in Chapter 5.

■ *If you are working out at a gym:* Choose three of the following machines for your cardio workout: elliptical trainer, treadmill, stationary bicycle, stepper. Stop to rest if you need to.

■ *If you are working out at home:* Use the cardio machine you have and train for 20 minutes without a break. *Or* take a brisk 15-minute walk outdoors, following my walking guidelines on pages 144–145. Stop to rest if you need to.

For the strength circuits

Perform the following exercises:

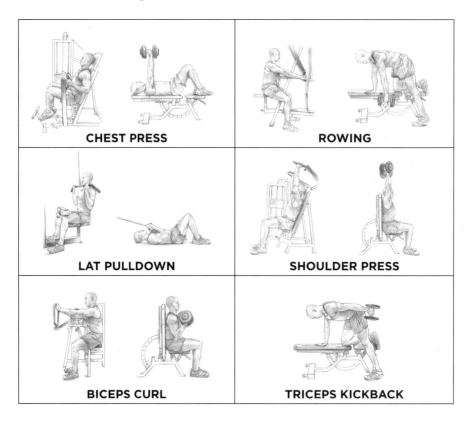

CHEST PRESS	ROWING
LAT PULLDOWN	SHOULDER PRESS
BICEPS CURL	TRICEPS KICKBACK

Follow the instructions on sets, repetitions, and maximum effort below. You may choose either version of each exercise, but I recommend the machine version and, if you're new to strength training, I recommend the machines. They place you in the correct posture automatically and help stabilize your body so that you don't get hurt.

In each of the three strength circuits, alternate sets of each exercise until you have completed all exercises and sets.

Cardio Circuit 1

Minutes 1–2: Using the cardio machine of your choice, press down on the bars or grips.

Minute 3: Push in, squeezing your chest muscles.

Minute 4: Pull out, squeezing your lat muscles.

Minutes 5–6: Press down, as in Minutes 1–2.

Strength Circuit 1

Perform 3 sets of 12 to 15 repetitions at 60 percent of your maximum effort, tweaking the intensity of your effort as necessary. Do not rest between sets.

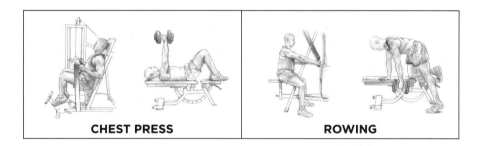

CHEST PRESS   **ROWING**

Cardio Circuit 2

If you are working out at a gym, switch to a different machine. Follow the guidelines for that machine (see Chapter 6, pages 140–43).

Minute 1: Using the cardio machine of your choice, press down on the bars or grips.

Minute 2: Push in, squeezing your chest muscles.

Minute 3: Pull out, squeezing your lat muscles.

Strength Circuit 2

Perform 3 sets of 12 to 15 repetitions at 60 percent of your maximum effort, tweaking the intensity of your effort as necessary. Do not rest between sets.

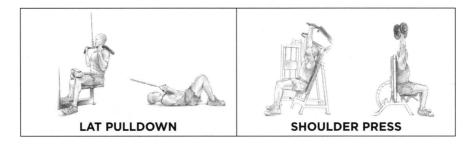

LAT PULLDOWN   **SHOULDER PRESS**

Cardio Circuit 3

Repeat Cardio Circuit 2. If you are working out at a gym, switch to a different machine. Follow the guidelines for that machine (see Chapter 6, pages 140–143).

Strength Circuit 3

Perform 3 sets of 12 to 15 repetitions at 60 percent of your maximum effort, tweaking the intensity of your effort as necessary. Do not rest between sets.

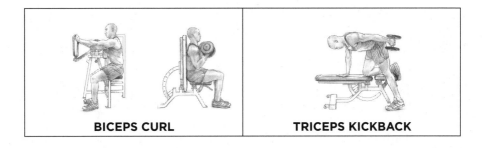

BICEPS CURL   **TRICEPS KICKBACK**

Cardio Circuit 4

Repeat Cardio Circuit 3. If you are working out at a gym, switch to a different machine. Follow the guidelines for that machine (see Chapter 6, pages 140–43).

Intermediate: Upper-Body Focus: Matwork

Do the Introductory mat (page 67) and/or the Beginner mat (page 83) until you can perform each exercise perfectly. Then graduate to the Intermediate mat, below. Remember your 3 C's—Concentration, Control, and Center—as well as Fluidity, Precision, and Breath.

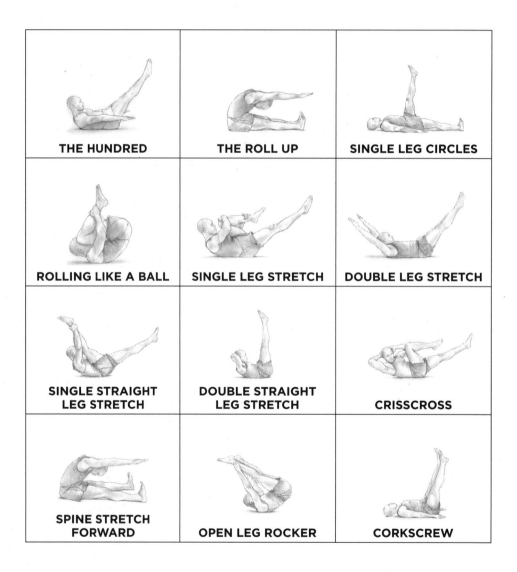

THE HUNDRED	THE ROLL UP	SINGLE LEG CIRCLES
ROLLING LIKE A BALL	SINGLE LEG STRETCH	DOUBLE LEG STRETCH
SINGLE STRAIGHT LEG STRETCH	DOUBLE STRAIGHT LEG STRETCH	CRISSCROSS
SPINE STRETCH FORWARD	OPEN LEG ROCKER	CORKSCREW

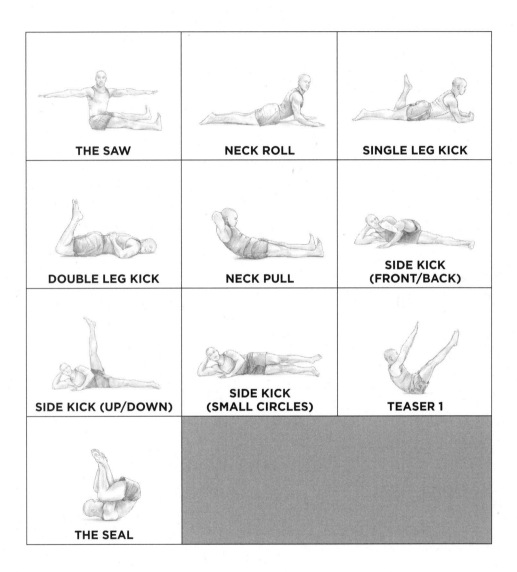

THE SAW	NECK ROLL	SINGLE LEG KICK
DOUBLE LEG KICK	NECK PULL	SIDE KICK (FRONT/BACK)
SIDE KICK (UP/DOWN)	SIDE KICK (SMALL CIRCLES)	TEASER 1
THE SEAL		

Cooldown: The Wall

Perform the Wall sequence in the order shown (see pages 132–135).

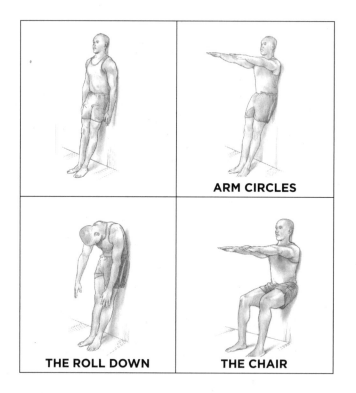

ARM CIRCLES

THE ROLL DOWN

THE CHAIR

14
SUCCESS STORIES

At the start of this program, maybe the first day, I gathered the group around me and told them the truth. "Achieving your goals will be a challenge," I said. "But it will also be doable." I added that they would get out of my program what they put in. Then we got to work.

Well, *they* got to work—and work they did. Their "after" photos, and the stories you're about to read, speak for themselves. I hope they inspire you, because there's no difference between them and you. If you work as hard as they did, you will be rewarded with a stronger, fitter body and a newfound lease on life.

It takes a strong mind to tell the body what to do, and a strong body to do what the mind asks. In the beginning, it isn't always easy to give up the "old ways." At times, your mind may rebel and your body may ache. But not for long. In time, on the machines and on the mat, your body and mind will learn to work together.

As your body changes, so does your sense of possibility. What can you do with your newly fit body? Where can you take it? What can it accomplish? The choices are up to you.

Aristotle, the Greek philosopher, once said, "We are what we repeatedly do. Excellence, therefore, is not an act but a habit." In other words, success won't come to you. You must take the first step, like Christiane, Tim, Angela, Cindy, and Miguel. Their stories could be yours. I hope they inspire you as much as this extraordinary group of ordinary people inspired me.

Christiane, 31

POUNDS LOST: 20

For the first week or two, this program was hard for me. Every workout kicked my butt. Every single exercise left me exhausted. I couldn't breathe. I thought I was going to die. But since then, I've gotten stronger and have much more endurance.

Just recently, while a few members of the group changed into their workout clothes, Chris told the rest of us to take a couple laps to warm up. The first week I couldn't finish even one lap. But that day, I ran the whole lap. We jogged back, and the rest of the group wasn't ready, so Chris told us to take another lap. I'm like, *God, I just did it once. But okay. I'll try.* I finished three quarters of the second lap and walked the rest of the way. When I walked up, they *still* weren't ready, so Chris said to take a third lap. I made it slightly more than halfway through before I pooped out. I thought, *That's pretty damn good. I can actually breathe.*

I still don't have any long-term weight goals. It will take some time before I'm actually skinny again, so I just go day by day. My only goal, if you can call it that, is to get stronger every day, and to eat healthily.

I've changed the way I eat, for sure. I don't starve myself—I definitely eat to satisfy—but I eat less crap. I eat whole-wheat pitas instead of white bread. I order steak with a side of steamed veggies rather than a baked potato with butter and sour cream. If I eat Mexican food, I go for the black beans, not the refried beans. I never ate fruit before I started this program, and now I have at least a piece a day. My diet isn't perfect, but I really think about the food I put in my mouth now, which helps enormously.

What will keep me going? Everything. I still want to perform again. I want to get up in the morning, see my reflection in the mirror, and think, *Damn, I'm hot!* I want to fit into cuter clothes. I have a pair of size 14 pants that fit a year and a half ago lying on a chair in my bedroom. I look at them every morning, and I think *Soon. Soon you will fit.* My goal is to be who I used to be. I very much remember how it felt to be fit and feel good.

This program is the best thing that has happened to me in a very long time. I don't want it to end. The good news is, Chris said he'd train us for a while longer, so he can get some awesome photos of this once-fat chick who got her hot ass back.

Tim, 35

POUNDS LOST: 20

This program has affected every part of my life. Yes, I've lost weight, and that's a big change. I've always worn my clothing two sizes too big because I thought looser clothes made me look thinner. Now my pants and shirts are about four sizes too big. I had to make a few new holes in my belt, but soon I'll have to buy some shirts and jeans in smaller sizes.

So I've lost weight. I feel better physically, but I also feel better emotionally. When I wake up in the morning, I'm ready to get on with the day.

Before I started the program, I'd get out of bed kind of down or even depressed, so there's a real difference in my mood, and I have energy like you wouldn't believe.

My relationship with my kids has changed, too. My wife Cindy always played with them. I tried, but I wasn't always so good at it. I can see now that my weight held me back. I remember huffing and puffing, pouring sweat, as I put a train set together. Now I can get down on the floor with the kids with no problems. We play board games. We hike. We go to the park. We interact more. I think I'm just a lot more fun for them.

Losing weight has also changed the way I see myself. Last year I tried out for the San Diego adult baseball league, which is a very competitive hardball league. I didn't make any of the teams, so I put together a team of all the other guys who didn't get picked. We called ourselves The Outlaws. We didn't win one game—we went 0 for 23, I think. That season I was always in a bad mood, and my shins hurt all the time.

This past spring I tried out for the league again. We'd been working out with Chris for about four and a half weeks. Cindy said to me, "I don't think you should try out this year. I don't want to go through this again." I said, "No, I'm trying out." I just wanted to see if I could get picked.

I did. Not only did I make a team, it was a team in the division higher than the league that I played in last year. I've been to just a few practices so far this year, and the difference in my performance compared to my performance last year is just amazing. It's like I've rediscovered my body and what it can do.

All this, just from eating better and working out a few days a week. Now that the program is over, I do Chris's cardio 30 minutes a day, three times a week, and play baseball. Cindy and I still cook healthy dinners together—we're not big fish people, so it's grilled chicken and steak, a little portion of brown rice, and lots of veggies. We just tried bulgur the other week, and Cindy just bought lentils to try. We keep each other motivated, which is one of the best parts of all this. I think losing weight as a couple has brought us closer. Our whole family is closer.

Angela, 30

POUNDS LOST: 18

I love this program. I've lost a bunch of weight, wear cuter clothes, and my muscles are stronger. I didn't expect that the program would improve my coordination, too, but that's a big plus, because I'm not the most coordinated person in the world.

In the first week of the program Chris showed the group how to do a certain exercise. To help us assume the proper form, he asked us to engage our core, then imagine holding a barrel. Then we were supposed to move back and forth. I thought I was doing a fabulous job until Chris checked on me. I couldn't hold the barrel without moving my hips like a salsa dancer. He had to stand behind me and hold me still. We all cracked up, even Chris. I can do that exercise now, though.

I still follow Chris's dietary guidelines, too—most of the time. I eat very little white sugar or white flour, but lots of lean chicken and fruit and beans. I had that binge at the restaurant opening, which I forgave myself for, but was able to do damage control and just go back to my healthy diet. Since then, I've done pretty well. I train too hard to mess up with the diet.

Chris said he will train us for a while more. We actually begged him to stick around because we've all done so well. This is great, because my goal is to get into even better shape for an upcoming vacation.

A few months back, my girlfriends and I decided to take a trip. We narrowed it down to two choices: lounge in the Greek islands or hike the Inca

Trail in Peru to see Machu Picchu, the Lost City of the Incas. We drew out of a hat. I was so excited when we picked Peru. I love to hike, and it's always been my dream to see Machu Picchu. I never had anyone to go with, and I'm not the type of person who takes a trip like that by myself.

But we really need to train for this trip. You can't be out of shape when you go to Machu Picchu—the place is almost 8,000 feet above sea level. It would be impossible to breathe at that high of an altitude. Many people take oxygen masks with them. Plus, I have asthma, which makes this goal even more of a challenge. I would be really upset to have flown to Peru and not get to see what I went there to see.

These workouts have definitely improved my endurance level, but I'm nowhere near ready. But if I continue with this program, I'll get there.

Oh, I almost forgot—I can paint my own toenails now! Yay! Although now that I know I can polish them without it being a workout in itself, I think I'll go back to getting pedicures.

Cindy, 44

POUNDS LOST: 10

I still have weight to lose, but for the first time in my life, I know that I can. In six weeks I learned what you need to do to lose weight. You actually have to eat—rather than starve yourself—and you have to move. That's all it takes, and it's very doable.

I love that I've lost weight, but the benefits of this program run deeper for me. My husband, Tim, mentioned that this plan has brought us closer as a family, and it's true. We do so much more with the kids. We used to take them shopping. Now we take hikes or go to the park. It's not just that Tim and I are more active. Our kids are, too, and that's a great thing.

I have more energy. I used to drink three or four cups of coffee in the morning, and two or three more in the afternoon. Now I drink one cup in the morning, and that's it. I drink less coffee, but have more energy. Who would have thought?

Though I'm not yet at my goal weight, my body has changed. My clothes are looser, because I've gained muscles and muscle takes up less space than fat. My arms are more defined, and I can feel my abdominal muscles. I know that if I stick to the program, I'll actually get to see them.

My posture has improved, and so has my coordination. At our first class, Chris had us stand on one leg, and I couldn't do it. He had to steady me. Now, I can balance on one foot as I hold a heavy medicine ball over my head. The program didn't just improve my core strength. It also improved my balance, which is an important part of fitness.

Tim and I still cook dinner together, and it's still fun. You just have to keep an open mind and be willing to try new foods. I watched a show recently, and the chef topped lentils with slices of filet mignon, and topped that with a yogurt sauce. It looked really good. I thought, *Heck, I can put steak on lentils.* So we've decided to try that dish.

We're going on vacation to Cabo San Lucas in a few months, and I don't want to go fat, like I did last time. I'd like to lose maybe 30 more pounds before our trip, so although our group workouts are over, I'll continue the program with Tim. For the first time in my life, I didn't go on some weird diet for a month and then say, "Thank God it's over." This is my life now—our life. We eat better, we incorporate exercise into our lives, and it's just a part of the routine, like brushing your teeth.

For those who are thinking about trying Chris's program, I'd say, once you start, stick with it. You will see results. Your body will change. Your life might even change—mine did. I always hated working out—if I did try to exercise, I'd go to one class, then quit. Not this time. I can see myself sticking to this program for the rest of my life.

Miguel, 32

POUNDS LOST: 10

My body has changed dramatically in a month and a half. It's like a total transformation. My upper body is extremely toned, but my midsection has improved the most. I can actually see my abdominals. I haven't had a six-pack since I was 17, and I love it.

Last weekend my family and parents and I all went to a restaurant. I wore a white T-shirt, and they all noticed my belly was gone. That was a great moment. They all laugh at me now, my wife especially, because I show off a little.

I don't just look better, I feel better. My body used to be very stiff, especially my back and shoulders—that's what happens when you sit at a desk virtually all day. Even though I hardly moved all day, I still needed eight to nine hours of sleep a night. The aches and stiffness are gone, and I wake up automatically after seven hours. My energy is through the roof. I can get through a long day, then go and work out. It's really true that the fitter you are, the more energy you have.

I also have more self-confidence. I wear a suit and tie maybe three times a week, and I was very self-conscious about my belly because it hung over my belt. My clients have noticed that I've lost weight and compliment me on how fit I look. That's definitely a positive.

To lose this weight, I really had to change my attitude about exercise and food. After just a few weeks on the program, I realized that I didn't miss my old way of life. I still don't. I think that most people who go on rigorous diets and workouts transform their life—for two months. Then they fall off the wagon because they could not stick to such a strict program for the rest of their lives. You don't feel like you have to sacrifice or miss out. You can live with this program.

Here's an example: I belong to a wine club—we meet once a month. Recently, the club hosted a dinner at one of my favorite restaurants, which serves very high-end Mexican cuisine. I ordered my red wine. I had my red meat—filet mignon instead of porterhouse, because it's a leaner cut.

For dessert, the restaurant served *crepas de cajeta*. This happens to be my favorite dessert. Probably I could have eaten it all, but I thought, *I have a workout tomorrow.* So I asked a friend for a bite of his. Just that spoonful satisfied me. If you eat well, you train better. When you train well, you tend to eat well, and vice versa. That's what Chris calls a positive spiral.

This way of life is my way of life now, for good. I run three or four times a week and joined a gym to keep up with the workouts Chris taught us. I'll stick with the food plan, for sure—easy on the processed foods, white sugar, and white flour. In six weeks, Chris gave me the foundation of an entirely new lifestyle that I've grown to love.

APPENDIX A:
BRINGING YOUR TRAINING TO LIFE

As a Pilates instructor, I tend to study people's posture as I walk around the city. They slump sideways into their hips with all their weight on one leg. They hunch over laptops in bookstores. They let their abdominals protrude, which throws their spines out of whack. I bet they feel the effects of their less-than-perfect posture by the end of the day in the form of neck, shoulder, and lower-back pain.

Although I've been an athlete all my life, I used to have terrible posture. I stood with my head cocked to one side, my arms across my chest, and all my weight on one leg. That changed when I met Romana.

The first time I met her—I was about to take my first class—she looked me up and down. Then she said, "Stand up straight. Pull your stomach in. Uncross your arms. Straighten your head and pull your chin in." I thought I looked cool, but Romana was like, turn the coolness down and *align*.

Core training doesn't end when you finish your workout. You need to bring the principles and concepts you practice there into your everyday life. Correct posture—keeping each body part in alignment with its adjacent parts—reflects core strength and stability. It stabilizes and protects the spine, and makes you appear more poised and confident. And because you're using your muscles more efficiently, your body actually needs less energy just to stand up straight—allowing you to meet the demands of your day with full force. Proper posture also places your lungs and other internal organs in the right position, so they function more effectively.

It's important to learn to attain and maintain correct posture in a variety of positions. I've chosen three of the most common: standing, sitting at a workstation, and going up and down stairs.

These corrections may not feel natural at first, but stick with them. Poor posture results from repeated patterns of movement, and so does proper posture. Correct those bad patterns—slouching, slumping, hunched shoulders—as soon as you notice them. Eventually you'll align and correct automatically.

STANDING

Think of each vertebra of your spine as a block, and your spinal column as a stack of blocks. Stack those blocks right on top of each other.

Hold your head up, elongate your neck, tuck your chin in, and look straight ahead. Lift your chest and press your shoulders back and away from your ears. Activate your powerhouse—engage your abdominals and contract your glutes. Lengthen through your waist and keep your knees soft. You should be able to draw a straight line from your ear through your shoulder, hip, knee, and ankle.

Correct Posture: Standing

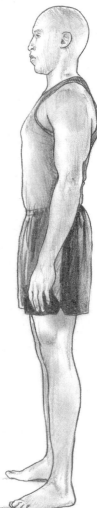

Assume Pilates stance

Square your Pilates box

Scoop

Elongate your neck and tuck your chin in

Press your shoulders back and down

Lengthen through your waist

Keep your knees soft

Contract your glutes

SITTING AT A WORKSTATION

Many of my clients have desk jobs. Even if they hadn't told me, I could have guessed by looking at their shoulders. Some of them actually had one shoulder higher than the other because they constantly cradled a phone between their ear and neck as they talked.

Sit in a chair with a back, if possible, and use the back support as a guide for proper spinal alignment. Sit with your entire back against the seat and activate your core. Place both feet on the floor. Do not sink into your lower back or cross your legs—both place stress on the lower back.

If your workstation has a computer, place the upper part of your monitor at eye level. Don't cradle the phone between your ear and neck—if you're always on the phone, ask for a headset. Try to leave your desk every 20 minutes to stretch your muscles and lengthen your spine.

CORRECT POSTURE: SITTING AT A WORK STATION

Thighs, hips, and knees form 90-degree angles

Square your Pilates box

Activate your core

Elongate your neck and tuck chin in

Press shoulders back and down

Contract your glutes—squeeze and grow tall

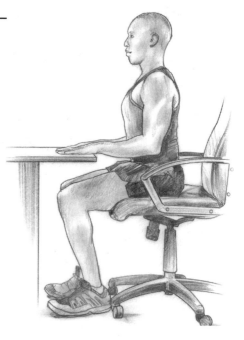

Climbing Stairs

Think of climbing stairs as standing in motion. As you ascend the stairs, contract your abdominal muscles to engage your glutes, and use your glutes to propel you forward and up. By the way, it's fine to bounce up the stairs, or to take stairs two at a time—as long as you're using your abs and glutes to propel you forward.

When you descend stairs, maintain correct alignment and use your stomach and glutes to decelerate.

Correct posture: Ascending and Descending Stairs

Contract abdominals and glutes to accelerate and decelerate

Elongate your neck and tuck chin in

Square your Pilates box

Keep your shoulders back and down

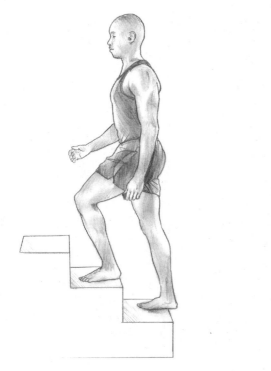
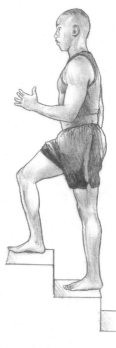

APPENDIX B:
TRAINING LOG

Photocopy pages 243–44 for extra training logs.

Date and time of workout _____

Hours of sleep _____

Today's weight _____

WORKOUT

Total-Body Focus

❏ Beginner

❏ Intermediate

Lower-Body Focus

❏ Beginner

❏ Intermediate

Upper-Body Focus

❏ Beginner

❏ Intermediate

Cardio

Machine Used	Time	Resistance	Speed
Treadmill			
Elliptical			
Bicycle			
Stepper			

Total cardio workout time _____

Intensity level (Borg scale) _____

Notes _____

_____

Strength

Exercises completed

Upper Body	Sets	Weight	Repetitions
Chest Press			
Rowing Machine			
Shoulder Press			
Biceps Curl			
Triceps Extensions			

Lower Body	Sets	Weight	Repetitions
Lunges			
Leg Extensions			
Leg Curls			
Hip Adduction			
Hip Abduction			
Calf Raise			

Notes _____

_____

Pilates

❑ Introductory mat ❑ Beginner mat ❑ Intermediate mat

Notes _____

_____

Mood

Mood before workout _____

Mood after workout _____

Thoughts/feelings during workout (mental focus, motivation level, etc.)

_____

Milestones

❑ Daily goal met ❑ Short-term goal met ❑ Long-term goal met

Personal best _____

ACKNOWLEDGMENTS

So many people helped create this book. I couldn't have done it without their guidance, talent, and support, and would like to extend a sincere thank-you.

Thanks to my friends and family—Robert, Dorothy, Michael, and Marcus—for their unfailing support and encouragement; my clients, for trusting me to help them achieve their fitness goals; and Saekson Jinjira, who taught me to train with heart.

I am also indebted to my many Pilates instructors; I learned from each one of you. Special thanks to Michael Johnson, for introducing me to the Method; Cynthia Shipley, for my weekly sessions; Inelia Garcia, for her discipline; Moses Urbano, for his technical advice; Jay Grimes, Sari Mejia Santo, and Romana Kryzanowska, for their lifelong dedication to preserving the Joseph Pilates work.

I am also extremely grateful to Paul Body, who so ably captured movement in the lens of a camera, and William Arbizu, who transformed Paul's photographs into the elegant illustrations within these pages.

To Kathi Ross-Nash, thanks for kicking my butt (in a good way). Thanks, too, to Jon Hines, for opening my eyes.

A final "thank-you" to my agent, Jan Miller, whose expert guidance helped shape this book, and the entire Simon Spotlight team.

ABOUT THE AUTHOR

A native of Houston, Chris Robinson is an elite personal trainer whose clients include celebrities, athletes, and top executives on both coasts. A lifelong athlete, Robinson is a two-time Muay Thai kickboxing champion and ran track and field at San Diego State University, where he earned a degree in kinesiology. He is also a certified Pilates instructor, and studied with the legendary Romana Kryzanowska, who learned the craft from Joseph Pilates himself.

Robinson is the founder and president of Core Coach Center, Inc.™ (www.corecoach.net), based in La Jolla, California.